The Complete Guide to Forgotten Home Apothecary

1000+ Timeless Remedies to Restore Your Health Naturally!

Rohit Sahu

Published by Rohit Sahu

Illustrations by: Pexels, Unsplash, Pixabay, Freepik (royalty-free image sources)

This book is a work of the author's research, experience, and knowledge of herbal remedies. The information provided is intended solely for educational and informational purposes and is not a substitute for professional medical advice, diagnosis, or treatment. Always consult with a qualified healthcare provider or herbalist before using any herbs or remedies, especially if you are pregnant, nursing, taking medications, or have an existing medical condition.

First Edition, 2024

Content

The Beginning of a Journey

As I sit down to write this note, I'm reminded of the winding path that led me here. The journey to create this book has been as much about rediscovering myself as it has been about collecting ancient herbal wisdom. From countless late nights researching remedies to moments of awe while walking in nature, this book is the culmination of years of learning, experimenting, and connecting with the timeless art of healing.

I didn't just want to create a book of recipes; I wanted to create a guide—a companion for anyone seeking a deeper connection to themselves, their loved ones, and the earth. Writing this has been a labor of love, an effort to make the vast and magical world of herbalism approachable and accessible to everyone, whether you're just beginning or looking to expand your knowledge.

If this book inspires you to brew your first cup of calming tea, soothe a little one's fever with a home remedy, or even just pause to appreciate the plants growing in your backyard, then I will consider this journey a success.

And if you find joy in these pages or if a remedy resonates with you, I'd be so grateful if you could share your thoughts. A kind review helps this book—and the love and care poured into it—reach others who might benefit from its wisdom. But most importantly, it lets me know how this book has touched your life, and that's the greatest gift of all.

Thank you for taking this step with me. May your apothecary always be abundant, and your spirit always grounded.

With gratitude and light,

Rohit 🌿

Part I: The Forgotten Art of Home Apothecary

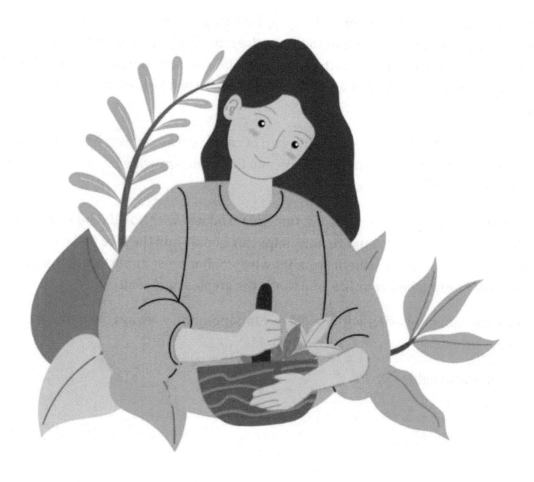

"Let food be thy medicine, and medicine be thy food." – Hippocrates

1.1 Rediscovering the Apothecary Tradition

In the fast-paced hum of modern life, where the glow of screens often overshadows the flicker of candlelight, we've lost touch with something profound: the quiet wisdom of the earth. For thousands of years, our ancestors turned to nature for answers, finding comfort in the roots, leaves, and flowers that grew around them. Their apothecaries weren't found in sterile aisles of pharmacies but in their gardens, forests, and kitchens—small, sacred spaces where healing began with the land itself.

As an Ayurvedic author and a student of ancient wisdom for over eight years, I've always been fascinated by how people cared for their health before pharmacies became the norm. Growing up, I would hear stories from my family about how remedies were made at home—simple, practical, and rooted in tradition.

I remember the way my mother would instinctively reach for fresh ginger when someone had a cough or how my father kept a small jar of neem oil for cuts and scrapes. It wasn't a formal apothecary, but it was a practice of relying on what was available in nature—without fanfare, but with deep trust in its effectiveness.

There was no mystery about it; it wasn't treated like magic. These remedies were just part of life—rituals of care and common sense that had been passed down over generations. It's this quiet, enduring knowledge that drew me to Ayurveda and the study of natural healing: the idea that wellness isn't something external to us but something we can nurture with the simplest tools.

Today, I realize how extraordinary that approach truly was. At its core, it wasn't about fancy equipment or obscure ingredients—it was about understanding the relationship between the body and the plants around us. That's what a home apothecary represents: empowerment through nature, simplicity, and connection to an ancient rhythm of living.

The Rise of Natural Healing in the Modern World

In recent years, we've witnessed a quiet yet undeniable revolution: a return to natural healing. It's not just a trend; it's a recognition that many of the answers we seek for our well-being don't lie in synthetic solutions but in the ancient harmony of nature.

As modern medicine advanced, we gained much—but we also lost something priceless. The home apothecary, once an essential part of every household, was relegated to history books. Yet, in this era of mass production and chemical dependency, people are beginning to ask: *What did we leave behind?*

The truth is, natural healing never disappeared; it was simply waiting for us to rediscover it. From the rise of organic farming to the popularity of mindfulness and holistic wellness, humanity is reconnecting with the earth in ways we couldn't have imagined a few decades ago. Today, making your own remedies isn't just a nod to the past; it's an act of empowerment.

What Is a Home Apothecary, and Why Does It Matter Today?

A home apothecary is more than a collection of jars and herbs—it's a philosophy. It's about taking control of your well-being, connecting with the natural world, and embracing the idea that healing can be simple, accessible, and deeply personal.

Imagine having the tools to soothe a sore throat with a honey and ginger infusion, calm an anxious mind with a lavender and chamomile tea, or brighten your skin with a calendula salve you made yourself. A home apothecary allows you to reclaim that knowledge and make your health a conversation between you and nature—not just a prescription pad.

But the value of a home apothecary goes beyond practicality. In a world that often feels disconnected and rushed, creating remedies with your own hands can be grounding and meditative. It's a way of saying, *I see you, nature. I trust you. I'm grateful for your gifts.*

This practice also carries the power to deepen family connections. When you teach your children or loved ones how to make remedies, you pass down something more than recipes—you pass down a legacy of care and self-reliance.

Stories of Herbal Wisdom Passed Down Through Generations

Herbal wisdom isn't just science; it's storytelling. It's the wisdom of grandmothers, healers, and farmers who observed the rhythms of the earth and shared their findings through tales and traditions. Every culture has its own herbal heritage, and these stories remind us that natural healing is universal.

I once heard the tale of a healer in a small Indian village who saved lives during a flu outbreak, not with fancy equipment but with turmeric milk infused with black pepper. She called it "golden protection," and the recipe was passed down from her ancestors. Similarly, in the Appalachian Mountains, elderberry syrup became a household staple to ward off colds and boost immunity—a practice that modern science now supports.

Even in times of war, herbal knowledge proved indispensable. During the Civil War in America, surgeons used calendula and yarrow to treat wounds on the battlefield. These plants, humble and unassuming, became lifesavers when modern supplies ran dry.

For me, the most profound stories are the personal ones. I'll never forget when I fell ill with COVID during the height of the pandemic. It was a time of uncertainty, fear, and debates over vaccines. My family and I, cautious about the side effects some people reported after vaccination, chose to lean on what we knew best: natural ways to support our health.

When the fever hit, and the body aches felt unbearable, it was my mother who stepped in, calm as always. Armed with nothing but garlic, honey, and a few other kitchen staples, she made a concoction that, to this day, I swear brought me back to life. She crushed fresh garlic cloves, stirred them into raw honey, and paired it with turmeric tea infused with a pinch of black pepper. It was simple yet powerful, and over the next few days, it became my lifeline.

It wasn't just the remedies that stayed with me—it was the way she used them. There was no panic, no second-guessing, just quiet confidence in the traditions she had inherited. It was a moment that reminded me of the power of ancestral wisdom: the idea that healing doesn't always have to come in complicated forms; sometimes, it's as simple as trusting nature.

That experience solidified my belief in the timelessness of natural remedies. It's one of the reasons I write— because these stories, these practices, are too valuable to lose. They represent a legacy that goes beyond generations. Writing this book is my way of preserving that legacy and sharing it with anyone willing to rediscover the ancient rhythm of natural healing.

The Call to Rediscover

What you hold in your hands is more than a book. It's an invitation to join a timeless tradition, to connect with the earth in a way that feels both ancient and revolutionary. This isn't about replacing modern medicine; it's about complementing it, enriching it with the gentle, restorative power of plants.

So, as you turn the pages, I encourage you to approach this journey with curiosity and gratitude. Imagine yourself as a modern herbalist, part scientist and part storyteller, rediscovering the lost art of the home apothecary.

Let's begin this journey together, one remedy at a time.

1.2 The Benefits of Herbal Remedies

Modern medicine has its place, no doubt—it saves lives and treats acute conditions with remarkable speed. But for everyday ailments like a lingering cough, restless sleep, or dry skin, store-bought solutions often come with a hidden cost.

- **Side Effects**: Many over-the-counter and prescription medications bring unwanted side effects, like drowsiness, digestive upset, or dependency. Natural remedies, when used responsibly, tend to be gentler on the body. For example, instead of using a chemical-laden cough syrup, a homemade ginger-honey tea can soothe a sore throat without any additives.
- **Empowerment**: Making your own remedies gives you control over what you put in your body. You know every ingredient, where it came from, and how it was prepared. There's something deeply empowering about turning to your kitchen or garden instead of a pill bottle.
- **Cost-Effective**: Store-bought medicines can be expensive, especially for recurring issues like allergies or digestive discomfort. A simple chamomile tea for sleep costs pennies compared to synthetic sleep aids—and it comes with none of the grogginess.
- **Sustainability**: Herbal remedies align with eco-conscious living. By growing, foraging, or sourcing local herbs, you reduce the environmental footprint of production, packaging, and shipping that accompanies store-bought products.

Understanding Holistic Wellness: Mind, Body, and Soul

When we think of health, we often focus solely on the body. But true wellness goes beyond physical health; it includes the mind and soul as well. This interconnected approach is at the heart of herbal medicine and holistic wellness.

1. Healing the Body

Herbal remedies often work by supporting the body's natural processes rather than suppressing symptoms. For example:

- **Immune Support**: Herbs like elderberry and echinacea don't just mask cold symptoms; they strengthen your immune system so you recover faster.
- **Digestive Health**: Instead of dulling stomach discomfort with antacids, remedies like ginger or peppermint work to ease inflammation and improve digestion naturally.
- **Skin Healing**: A calendula salve doesn't just sit on the surface—it promotes cell regeneration and reduces irritation.

Unlike many synthetic medicines, which target a specific symptom, herbs often have a broad spectrum of benefits, improving overall health while addressing the root cause.

2. Nurturing the Mind

In our busy lives, mental health often takes a back seat. But herbal remedies can provide much-needed support:

- **Stress Relief**: Adaptogens like ashwagandha and holy basil help balance cortisol levels, reducing the long-term effects of stress.
- **Better Sleep**: Lavender, chamomile, and valerian root can calm the nervous system, helping you unwind without the side effects of synthetic sleep aids.

Herbal remedies are often used as part of rituals—making tea, lighting a candle, or massaging oil into the skin—which creates a sense of mindfulness and intentionality that soothes the mind.

3. Connecting with the Soul

There's something deeply spiritual about using plants for healing. Growing, harvesting, and preparing remedies connects you to the natural world in a way that feels grounding and sacred. It reminds us that we're part of something larger—that the earth provides for us when we care for it in return.

Even small rituals, like steeping tea or inhaling the aroma of a lavender sprig, can foster a sense of calm and gratitude. This connection nourishes not just the body but the spirit, making herbal medicine a truly holistic practice.

The Science Behind How Herbal Medicine Works

For those who wonder if herbal remedies are "real medicine," it's worth noting that many modern drugs are derived from plants. Herbal medicine has been around for thousands of years, and its efficacy is increasingly supported by scientific research.

1. The Chemistry of Healing

Plants contain active compounds—like alkaloids, flavonoids, tannins, and essential oils—that interact with the body in powerful ways. For example:

- **Turmeric**: The curcumin in turmeric is a potent anti-inflammatory, often used to ease arthritis and digestive issues.
- **Peppermint**: Its menthol content relaxes muscles in the digestive tract, relieving bloating and gas.

- **Garlic**: Rich in allicin, garlic is a natural antibacterial and antifungal agent, useful for fighting infections.

Unlike synthetic drugs, which often isolate a single compound, herbal remedies use the whole plant. This allows the various compounds to work synergistically, enhancing their effectiveness and reducing side effects.

2. Supporting the Body, Not Overpowering It

Herbal remedies encourage the body to heal itself rather than forcing a reaction. For example:

- Adaptogens like rhodiola and ashwagandha help the body regulate stress hormones rather than simply masking the symptoms of stress.
- Herbal teas like ginger and fennel stimulate the digestive system, promoting balance rather than just dulling discomfort.

3. Evidence Meets Tradition

Many herbal remedies are supported by both traditional use and modern science. For example:

- Elderberry syrup, long used as a folk remedy for colds, has been shown in studies to reduce the duration and severity of flu symptoms.
- Chamomile tea, a centuries-old sleep aid, contains apigenin, a compound that binds to receptors in the brain to promote relaxation.

This intersection of science and tradition highlights the enduring power of herbal medicine.

Choosing herbal remedies isn't about rejecting modern medicine—it's about complementing it with practices that are gentle, empowering, and deeply connected to nature. It's about embracing a philosophy of healing that sees wellness not as a quick fix, but as a balance to be nurtured over time.

By understanding the benefits of herbal remedies, you're not just reclaiming ancient wisdom—you're also taking a step toward a more mindful, sustainable, and connected way of living.

1.3 The Basics of Herbal Healing

Herbal healing is both an art and a science, blending traditional wisdom with practical techniques that have been refined over centuries. To truly embrace the craft of creating remedies, it's essential to understand the different types of preparations, the subtle energetics of plants, and how herbs interact with the body to promote balance and healing. This chapter will guide you through the foundational principles that form the heart of natural healing.

Types of Herbal Remedies

Herbs can be transformed into a variety of preparations depending on the desired outcome and the parts of the plant being used. Each type of remedy has unique applications and benefits.

1. Teas and Infusions

What They Are: Water-based preparations made by steeping herbs in hot water, much like brewing tea.

Best For: Delicate plant parts like leaves and flowers (e.g., chamomile, peppermint).

How They Work: The heat of the water extracts water-soluble compounds, such as flavonoids and tannins, which are beneficial for calming the nervous system or aiding digestion.

Example:

- Chamomile tea for insomnia.
- Peppermint tea for indigestion.

2. Decoctions

What They Are: A more robust version of an infusion, made by simmering tougher plant parts like roots, bark, or seeds in water for an extended period.

Best For: Extracting compounds from harder materials (e.g., ginger root, cinnamon bark).

Example:

- Ginger decoction for nausea or colds.

3. Tinctures

What They Are: Alcohol-based extracts of herbs that preserve their active compounds for long-term use.

Best For: Potent, concentrated doses of medicinal herbs like echinacea or ashwagandha.

How They Work: Alcohol extracts both water- and fat-soluble compounds, making tinctures especially powerful and shelf-stable.

Example:

- Echinacea tincture for boosting immunity.

4. Salves and Balms

What They Are: Oil-based remedies thickened with beeswax to create a semi-solid form that's applied to the skin.

Best For: Wound healing, muscle pain, and dry skin.

How They Work: The fat-soluble compounds in herbs, like calendula or arnica, penetrate the skin to provide localized relief.

Example:

- Calendula salve for soothing cuts and rashes.

5. Herbal Oils

What They Are: Infused oils made by steeping herbs in a carrier oil (like olive or coconut oil) to extract their properties.

Best For: Massages, skincare, and as a base for salves.

Example:

- Lavender-infused oil for relaxation and minor burns.

6. Syrups

What They Are: Sweet, concentrated herbal preparations made by combining an herbal decoction or infusion with honey or sugar.

Best For: Coughs and soothing sore throats.

Example:

- Elderberry syrup for colds and flu.

7. Poultices and Compresses

What They Are: External applications of crushed herbs or soaked cloths, applied directly to the skin.

Best For: Drawing out toxins, soothing inflammation, and reducing swelling.

Example:

- Plantain poultice for insect bites.

8. Oxymels

What They Are: A blend of vinegar and honey infused with herbs.

Best For: Respiratory support and digestive health.

Example:

- Thyme oxymel for cough relief.

By understanding these different types of remedies, you'll have a toolkit to address a wide range of needs, whether you're soothing a cough, calming stress, or supporting your skin.

Understanding Plant Energetics

One of the most fascinating aspects of herbal healing is recognizing how plants carry energetic properties that influence the body. This concept is central to many traditional healing systems, including Ayurveda, Traditional Chinese Medicine, and Western herbalism.

1. Cooling Herbs

What They Do: Reduce heat, inflammation, or irritation in the body.

Best For: Fevers, skin rashes, hot flashes, or digestive heat (e.g., acid reflux).

Examples:

- **Peppermint**: Cools the digestive system and calms inflammation.
- **Cucumber**: A cooling herb for skin irritations or heat-related conditions.

2. Warming Herbs

What They Do: Stimulate circulation, increase warmth, and boost energy.

Best For: Cold hands and feet, sluggish digestion, or respiratory congestion.

Examples:

- **Ginger**: Warms the digestive system and relieves nausea.
- **Cinnamon**: Enhances circulation and warms the body during colds.

3. Moistening Herbs

What They Do: Add hydration and soothe dryness in tissues.

Best For: Dry skin, irritated mucous membranes, or chronic dehydration.

Examples:

- **Marshmallow root**: Soothes dry throats and digestive tracts.
- **Oats**: A moistening herb for dry skin or inflamed tissues.

4. Drying Herbs

What They Do: Reduce excess moisture, phlegm, or dampness in the body.

Best For: Wet coughs, swelling, or fungal conditions.

Examples:

- **Sage**: Dries excessive sweating and sore throats.
- **Yarrow**: Dries wounds and helps with damp skin conditions.

Understanding plant energetics allows you to choose herbs based on their effects, creating remedies that restore balance to the body.

An Overview of Herbal Actions

Herbs work through a variety of mechanisms, known as herbal actions, which describe how they influence the body. Here's a quick guide to some of the most common actions:

1. Anti-Inflammatory

What It Does: Reduces inflammation in the body.

Best For: Arthritis, muscle pain, or irritated skin.

Examples: Turmeric, ginger, calendula.

2. Antimicrobial

What It Does: Fights bacteria, viruses, or fungi.

Best For: Infections, colds, and wounds.

Examples: Garlic, thyme, tea tree oil.

3. Adaptogenic

What It Does: Helps the body adapt to stress and restores balance.

Best For: Chronic stress, fatigue, or hormonal imbalance.

Examples: Ashwagandha, holy basil, rhodiola.

4. Nervine

What It Does: Calms the nervous system and reduces anxiety.

Best For: Stress, insomnia, or tension headaches.

Examples: Chamomile, valerian, passionflower.

5. Astringent

What It Does: Tightens tissues and reduces secretions.

Best For: Diarrhea, wounds, or excessive sweating.

Examples: Witch hazel, sage, blackberry leaf.

6. Digestive

What It Does: Improves digestion, reduces bloating, and soothes the stomach.

Best For: Indigestion, gas, or sluggish digestion.

Examples: Peppermint, fennel, dandelion root.

7. Diaphoretic

What It Does: Promotes sweating to reduce fevers and detoxify the body.

Best For: Fevers, colds, or detoxification.

Examples: Elderflower, ginger, yarrow.

8. Demulcent

What It Does: Soothes and protects mucous membranes.

Best For: Dry throats, irritated skin, or ulcers.

Examples: Marshmallow root, aloe vera.

By understanding these actions, you can select herbs that match the specific needs of your body, creating remedies that are tailored, effective, and holistic.

The beauty of herbal healing lies in its diversity and depth. Whether you're sipping a calming tea, applying a soothing salve, or taking an adaptogenic tincture, every remedy is an opportunity to nurture balance in your body. By understanding the types of remedies, plant energetics, and herbal actions, you now have the foundation to create healing solutions that honor both tradition and your unique needs.

Join me in the next chapter as we explore how to build your confidence as a beginner, empowering you to start crafting remedies with ease and trust in your abilities.

1.4 Building Confidence as a Beginner

I know, the world of herbal medicine can feel overwhelming at first. With so much information out there, it's easy to second-guess yourself or feel intimidated by the process. But like any skill, herbal healing becomes second nature with time, practice, and a willingness to learn. This chapter is your guide to starting with confidence by addressing common myths, providing safety guidelines, and teaching you how to trust your body's signals.

Busting Myths About Herbal Medicine

There are plenty of misconceptions surrounding herbal remedies that can hold beginners back. Let's clear the air and debunk some of the most common myths.

Myth 1: Herbal Medicine Isn't Effective

Many people assume that natural remedies are less effective than pharmaceuticals because they work "too slowly." The truth is that herbs often work on a deeper level, addressing root causes rather than just masking symptoms. For example:

- **Chamomile tea** calms the nervous system and improves sleep quality over time, unlike over-the-counter sleep aids that can cause dependency.
- **Turmeric** reduces inflammation systemically, supporting long-term joint health rather than just providing short-term pain relief.

Myth 2: You Need a Lot of Experience to Use Herbs

It's easy to think you need to be an expert to start working with herbs. But herbal healing is deeply intuitive. You don't need a degree to make a cup of peppermint tea for an upset stomach or use aloe vera on a burn. Start simple, and let your confidence grow as you see the results.

Myth 3: Herbal Medicine Is Dangerous

When used responsibly, herbs are some of the safest tools for healing. Compared to synthetic medications, which often come with a long list of side effects, many herbs are gentle enough for everyday use. Safety comes down to understanding the proper dosages and knowing which herbs to avoid in certain situations (we'll cover this next).

Myth 4: All Natural Remedies Are Safe

While herbal medicine is generally safe, "natural" doesn't always mean harmless. Some plants can be toxic if misused or if taken in excessive amounts. For instance:

- **Foxglove** can be deadly if consumed.
- Herbs like **comfrey** are best used externally due to potential liver toxicity if ingested.

The key is research and moderation. When in doubt, stick to tried-and-true remedies with a long history of safe use.

Safety Guidelines for Using Herbs at Home

Safety is the foundation of herbal medicine, and following a few key principles ensures a positive experience.

1. Start Small and Go Slow

- Always introduce one herb or remedy at a time. This allows you to observe how your body reacts before combining it with other treatments.
- For teas, start with a mild dosage, such as 1 teaspoon of dried herb per cup of water, and increase gradually if needed.

2. Know Your Source

- Only use herbs from trusted suppliers to avoid contamination with pesticides, heavy metals, or other harmful substances.
- If foraging, ensure you properly identify plants before harvesting them. Many edible plants have toxic lookalikes (e.g., wild carrot vs. poison hemlock).

3. Be Aware of Allergies and Sensitivities

- Test a small amount of a new herb on your skin or as a diluted tea before using it extensively.
- Common allergic reactions include itching, redness, or mild swelling. Stop use immediately if you notice any adverse effects.

4. Avoid Certain Herbs During Pregnancy or Nursing

Some herbs can stimulate uterine contractions or pass through breast milk to your baby. Herbs to avoid include:

- **Pennyroyal** (can cause uterine stimulation).
- **Sage** (may reduce milk supply).
- Stick to gentle, well-known herbs like **ginger**, **chamomile**, and **raspberry leaf** (in moderation).

5. Understand Dosages

- Just like pharmaceuticals, herbs work best when taken in the right amounts. Always follow recommended guidelines for teas, tinctures, and other preparations.
- As a beginner, use reference books or online resources to check dosage recommendations.

6. Consult with Professionals

If you're on medications, always check for potential interactions. For example:

- **St. John's Wort** can interfere with antidepressants.
- **Gingko biloba** can thin the blood, increasing the risk of bleeding when combined with blood thinners.

Consult a qualified herbalist or healthcare provider before using herbs if you have a preexisting condition.

7. Label Everything

- Always label jars, bottles, and tins with the herb name, preparation date, and intended use. This prevents confusion and ensures you're using remedies within their shelf life.

How to Listen to Your Body and Track Remedies Effectively?

Your body is one of the best guides in herbal healing. Learning to observe how it responds to different herbs and remedies will help you refine your approach over time.

1. Notice the Subtle Changes

Herbal remedies often work gently, and their effects may take time to notice. Pay attention to:

- **Physical symptoms**: Do you feel less bloated after taking fennel tea? Is your cough improving after elderberry syrup?
- **Emotional responses**: Do calming herbs like chamomile or valerian help you relax?

2. Keep a Remedy Journal

Tracking your experiences helps you understand what works for your unique needs. Create a simple system for logging your remedies:

- **Date**: When you took the remedy.
- **Herb/Preparation**: What you used and how it was prepared (e.g., peppermint tea, ginger tincture).
- **Reason**: What symptom or issue you were addressing.
- **Outcome**: How you felt afterward.

Sample Entry:

- **Date**: March 10, 2024
- **Herb/Preparation**: Chamomile tea (1 tsp dried flowers, steeped 10 minutes).
- **Reason**: Trouble sleeping due to stress.
- **Outcome**: Felt calmer within 30 minutes, slept through the night.

Over time, patterns will emerge, giving you insight into which remedies best suit your body.

3. Respect Your Intuition

Your body often knows what it needs. If a certain remedy feels "off" or doesn't resonate, trust that feeling. Likewise, if you feel drawn to a particular herb, it may be worth exploring why.

4. Pay Attention to Dosage and Duration

- **Short-Term Use**: Some herbs, like elderberry, are best for acute conditions and shouldn't be taken daily for extended periods.
- **Long-Term Use**: Adaptogens like ashwagandha can be taken over weeks or months to build resilience.

Always take breaks from herbal remedies to allow your body to reset and avoid dependence.

Building Confidence Through Simplicity

One of the best ways to build confidence is to start small and keep things simple. Choose one or two herbs to work with initially—herbs that are versatile, safe, and easy to source, such as:

- **Chamomile**: Calming, aids digestion, and improves sleep.
- **Peppermint**: Soothes the stomach, clears sinuses, and relieves tension headaches.

Master a few simple remedies, like teas or infused oils, before exploring more advanced techniques. Confidence comes not from knowing everything at once, but from taking small, meaningful steps.

Trusting Yourself on This Journey

Building confidence as a beginner isn't about perfection—it's about trusting yourself to learn, experiment, and grow. Herbal medicine is a journey, not a destination, and every cup of tea or jar of salve you make brings you closer to mastering the art.

In the next chapters, you'll continue expanding your skills, diving into remedies that address common ailments, and discovering the joy of creating your own healing solutions. Take it one step at a time—confidence will follow.

Part II: Essentials for Your Home Apothecary

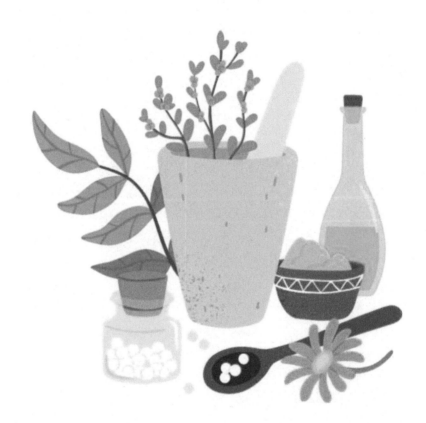

"For every human illness, somewhere in the world there exists a plant which is the cure." – Rudolf Steiner

2.1 Your Herbal Pantry

Building your herbal pantry is one of the most exciting steps in creating your home apothecary. It's about curating a collection of versatile, effective, and easy-to-use ingredients that will form the foundation of your remedies. Whether you're soothing a sore throat, calming the mind, or easing a skin irritation, these essentials will empower you to craft healing solutions with confidence.

Introduction to Beginner-Friendly Herbs

Herbs are the heart of any home apothecary, and some are especially suited for beginners due to their versatility, safety, and wide availability. Let's explore four cornerstone herbs that are both gentle and powerful:

1. Chamomile (Matricaria chamomilla)

Uses:

- Calms the nervous system, aids digestion, and promotes restful sleep.
- Soothes irritated skin when used in salves or compresses.

How to Use: Brew as a tea for relaxation or infuse into oil for skin remedies.

Fun Fact: Known as the "physician of the plants," chamomile enhances the growth of nearby herbs in a garden.

2. Peppermint (Mentha × piperita)

Uses:

- Eases digestive issues like bloating and indigestion.
- Relieves tension headaches and clears nasal congestion.

How to Use: Prepare as a tea for stomach discomfort or inhale steam infused with peppermint for sinus relief.

Fun Fact: Ancient Egyptians used peppermint in burial rituals and as a remedy for digestive ailments.

3. Calendula (Calendula officinalis)

Uses:

- Anti-inflammatory and antimicrobial properties make it ideal for cuts, scrapes, and burns.
- Promotes glowing, hydrated skin.

How to Use: Infuse into oils for salves or use dried petals in soothing teas.

Fun Fact: Calendula was historically used to dye fabrics and create golden-hued food dishes.

4. Lavender (Lavandula angustifolia)

Uses:

- Calms the mind, promotes sleep, and soothes irritated skin.
- Effective in balms, oils, and as a natural insect repellent.

How to Use: Add dried flowers to bath soaks, or create a calming linen spray with lavender essential oil.

Fun Fact: Lavender has been used in perfumery and medicine since ancient Roman times.

These four herbs are an excellent starting point, but they're just the beginning. As you grow more confident, you'll discover the beauty and benefits of dozens of other herbs that can become part of your apothecary.

20 Pantry Staples for a Well-Stocked Apothecary

Your herbal pantry isn't just about herbs. A complete apothecary includes foundational ingredients that allow you to create a wide range of remedies. Here are 20 essential staples to keep on hand:

Base Ingredients (Herbs and Powders)

1. **Dried Ginger**: A warming herb for nausea, colds, and circulation.
2. **Elderberries**: Rich in antioxidants and a key ingredient for immune-boosting syrups.
3. **Turmeric Powder**: An anti-inflammatory powerhouse for teas and tonics.
4. **Plantain Leaves**: Excellent for soothing bug bites and minor skin irritations.
5. **Marshmallow Root**: A moistening herb that soothes dry throats and irritated skin.

Sweeteners and Preservatives

6. **Raw Honey**: Antibacterial, soothing, and perfect for syrups, teas, and skin remedies.
7. **Apple Cider Vinegar**: An excellent base for tonics and oxymels that promote digestion and immunity.
8. **Alcohol (e.g., Vodka or Brandy)**: A key ingredient for tinctures, extracting and preserving herbal properties.

Carrier Oils

9. **Olive Oil**: A versatile oil for infusing herbs and making salves.
10. **Coconut Oil**: Antimicrobial and moisturizing, ideal for balms and skincare.
11. **Almond Oil**: Gentle and nourishing for sensitive skin remedies.

Essential Oils

12. **Lavender Essential Oil**: A calming, multi-purpose oil for stress relief and skin care.
13. **Tea Tree Essential Oil**: Antimicrobial and cleansing, perfect for acne and minor cuts.

Clays and Powders

14. **Bentonite Clay**: Draws out toxins and soothes irritated skin when used in masks or poultices.
15. **Arrowroot Powder**: A natural thickener for creams and salves.

Teas and Seeds

16. **Fennel Seeds**: A digestive aid and calming tea ingredient.
17. **Peppermint Leaves**: For teas and infused oils.

Miscellaneous Staples

18. **Epsom Salt**: A key ingredient for muscle-soothing bath soaks.
19. **Beeswax**: Used to solidify salves and balms.
20. **Cheesecloth or Muslin Bags**: For straining tinctures, syrups, and infusions.

With these staples in your pantry, you'll have everything you need to begin making teas, syrups, tinctures, salves, and more.

A Guide to Sourcing Herbs: Buying vs. Growing Your Own

One of the joys of building an apothecary is deciding how to source your herbs. Whether you choose to grow your own or purchase them, here's how to ensure you're working with the highest-quality ingredients:

Where to Shop:

- Look for trusted suppliers who specialize in organic or wildcrafted herbs. Examples include online retailers, local health food stores, or herbal apothecaries.
- Farmers' markets often offer fresh, locally grown herbs.

What to Look For:

- **Color and Aroma**: High-quality dried herbs retain vibrant colors and a strong scent. Avoid anything that looks faded or smells musty.
- **Packaging**: Choose herbs stored in airtight containers to preserve potency.
- **Cost-Saving Tip**: Buy in small quantities to start and expand your collection as needed. Bulk herbs can save money, but only if you use them before they lose potency.

Growing Your Own Herbs

Starting your own herb garden can be incredibly rewarding, even if you only have a small space.

Easy Herbs for Beginners:

- **Basil**: Great for digestion and culinary use.
- **Lemon Balm**: Calms the mind and promotes sleep.
- **Parsley**: Rich in nutrients and a gentle diuretic.

Where to Grow:

- Herbs thrive in well-drained soil with plenty of sunlight.
- If space is limited, try growing herbs in containers on a windowsill, balcony, or small patio.

Harvesting Tips:

- Pick herbs early in the morning, after the dew has dried but before the sun becomes too hot.
- Air-dry small bundles in a cool, dark place, then store in airtight containers for long-term use.

A well-stocked herbal pantry is the cornerstone of your home apothecary. By starting with versatile herbs like chamomile and lavender and pairing them with pantry staples like honey and olive oil, you'll have the tools to create a wide variety of remedies. Whether you choose to buy or grow your ingredients, remember that every jar and bottle you add to your collection is a step toward self-reliance and connection to nature.

In the next chapter, we'll explore the tools of the trade and how to set up an organized, functional apothecary space that suits your needs.

2.2 Tools of the Trade

Creating herbal remedies is a hands-on craft, and having the right tools can make all the difference. While you don't need an elaborate setup to start, investing in a few essential tools will help you craft effective and high-quality remedies with ease. This chapter will guide you through the tools you'll need and how to create a functional, organized apothecary space, whether you're working with a spacious kitchen or a single shelf.

Essential Tools for Herbal Remedy-Making

A good apothecary doesn't require fancy or expensive equipment—just practical tools that simplify the process of preparing, storing, and using herbal remedies. Below is a list of must-have tools, grouped by their purpose:

1. Preparation Tools

These tools help you chop, grind, and extract the active compounds from herbs.

1. Mortar and Pestle:

- **Use**: Crush fresh or dried herbs to release their oils and medicinal properties.
- **Why It's Essential**: A timeless tool for making herbal pastes, powders, or small-batch remedies.

2. Herb Scissors or Sharp Knife:

- **Use**: For finely chopping fresh herbs like basil, parsley, or rosemary.
- **Why It's Essential**: Ensures even extraction when preparing remedies like infusions or poultices.

3. Grater or Microplane:

- **Use**: To finely grate ginger, turmeric, or citrus peels for teas and tonics.

4. Cheesecloth or Muslin Bags:

- **Use**: For straining infusions, tinctures, and syrups.
- **Why It's Essential**: Keeps your remedies smooth and free from herb particles.

5. Digital Scale:

- **Use**: To measure herbs and ingredients accurately, especially for tinctures and salves.
- **Pro Tip**: Look for one that can measure small quantities (grams or ounces).

2. Cooking and Brewing Tools

These tools are essential for creating teas, decoctions, and infused oils.

1. Stainless Steel or Enamel Saucepan:

- **Use**: For simmering herbs when making decoctions, syrups, or herbal oils.
- **Why It's Essential**: Non-reactive surfaces preserve the integrity of the herbs.

2. Tea Kettle or French Press:

- **Use**: To brew herbal teas and infusions easily.
- **Why It's Essential**: A French press is especially useful for straining teas.

3. Double Boiler:

- **Use**: For gently heating oils when making salves or infusions.
- **Alternative**: Create a makeshift double boiler by placing a heatproof bowl over a pot of simmering water.

4. Thermometer:

- **Use**: To monitor temperatures for salves, syrups, and infused oils.
- **Pro Tip**: Choose one with a wide temperature range for versatility.

3. Storage and Application Tools

Your remedies will need proper containers and tools for application to stay fresh and effective.

1. Mason Jars (Various Sizes):

- **Use**: For infusions, tinctures, and storing dried herbs.
- **Why It's Essential**: They're airtight, reusable, and easy to sterilize.

2. Glass Bottles with Droppers:

- **Use**: For tinctures, oils, and herbal syrups.
- **Why It's Essential**: Droppers allow for precise dosing.

3. Tins or Small Jars:

- **Use**: For storing salves, balms, and creams.
- **Pro Tip**: Choose dark glass or metal tins to protect remedies from light exposure.

4. Spray Bottles:

- **Use**: For room sprays, facial mists, and herbal cleaning solutions.

4. Miscellaneous Tools

1. Funnels:

- **Use**: To transfer liquid remedies into bottles or jars without spilling.

2. Labels and Markers:

- **Use**: For writing the name of the remedy, ingredients, preparation date, and expiration date.
- **Why It's Essential**: Proper labeling ensures safety and prevents mix-ups.

3. Blender or Food Processor:

- **Use**: For making herbal pastes, powdered blends, or emulsifying creams.

4. Strainer or Fine Mesh Sieve:

- **Use**: To strain out herbs from infusions, decoctions, or tinctures.

5. Heatproof Glass Measuring Cups:

- **Use**: For measuring liquids or as small mixing bowls.

How to Set Up a Functional and Organized Apothecary Space

No matter your space constraints, a well-organized apothecary allows you to work efficiently and keep your remedies fresh. Here's how to create a functional setup that suits your needs:

1. Designate a Space

Choose a space that's convenient but out of direct sunlight to preserve the potency of your herbs and remedies.

- **Kitchen Cabinet or Pantry Shelf**: Ideal for beginners with limited space. Use stackable jars and baskets to keep things neat.
- **Dedicated Apothecary Corner**: For those with more room, a small cabinet or shelving unit can house your ingredients, tools, and books. Include hooks or bars to hang drying herbs.

2. Organize by Category

Group items by their purpose for easier access.

- **Herbs**: Store dried herbs in airtight jars labeled with the name, date, and origin. Keep them grouped by function (e.g., digestive aids, calming herbs).
- **Tools**: Dedicate a drawer or basket for strainers, scissors, and funnels.
- **Containers**: Arrange jars, bottles, and tins by size on a separate shelf.

3. Maximize Freshness

Proper storage is key to maintaining the quality of your herbs and remedies.

- **Light Protection**: Store herbs in amber or dark glass containers to block light, which can degrade their potency.
- **Cool and Dry**: Choose a space with low humidity and a stable temperature. Avoid storing herbs near a stove or oven.
- **Rotation**: Use older herbs first to avoid waste. Most dried herbs retain their potency for 6–12 months.

4. Personalize Your Space

Add touches that make your apothecary inviting and inspiring:

- Include a small chalkboard or whiteboard to write down experiments or reminders.
- Add books or journals for quick reference or note-taking.
- Decorate with dried herb bundles, small potted plants, or vintage jars for a rustic feel.

A Day in Your Apothecary

Imagine stepping into your apothecary corner. You pull a jar of chamomile from the shelf, measure it carefully into a French press, and pour boiling water over it to steep. While the tea brews, you reach for a bottle of lavender-infused oil to soothe your dry hands. Every tool, herb, and jar is within reach, making the process seamless and enjoyable.

This is the beauty of an organized apothecary—it transforms the process of creating remedies into a ritual of self-care and empowerment. With the right tools and a thoughtfully arranged space, your home apothecary becomes a sanctuary for healing and creativity. Every jar, bottle, and strainer you add is an investment in your journey toward natural wellness.

2.3 Growing Your Own Apothecary Garden

Growing your own herbs has always felt like a grounding ritual to me—a way to connect with nature in its simplest, most intimate form. I'll never forget the first time I planted chamomile in a small terracotta pot on my windowsill. At the time, I didn't have a garden or much experience with plants, but watching those tiny seeds sprout into delicate flowers felt like witnessing a small miracle. The first cup of tea I made with those blossoms was more than soothing; it was transformative. It wasn't just tea—it was something I had nurtured with my own hands.

Of course, I understand that not everyone has the luxury of space for a full garden, and that's perfectly fine. You don't need sprawling fields or even a backyard to grow healing herbs. A windowsill, a balcony, or even a corner of your living room can be enough to start small. But for those who *do* have the opportunity to cultivate a garden, I can't recommend it enough. There's a kind of magic in walking out to harvest lavender for a calming oil or clipping fresh mint for a digestive tea. It's not just about the remedies you create—it's about the connection you build with the earth and the self-reliance that comes with it.

In this chapter, I'll guide you through the process of creating your own apothecary garden, whether it's a single pot or a thriving herb bed.

Easy-to-Grow Medicinal Plants for Small Spaces

Whether you have a full garden, a small patio, or just a sunny windowsill, you can grow these beginner-friendly medicinal plants:

1. Chamomile (Matricaria chamomilla)

Why Grow It: Chamomile is a gentle herb for calming nerves, promoting sleep, and soothing the skin.

How to Grow:

- Grows well in pots or garden beds with full sun.
- Prefers well-drained, sandy soil.

Harvesting: Pick the daisy-like flowers when fully open and dry them for teas and infusions.

2. Mint (Mentha spp.)

Why Grow It: Peppermint or spearmint is excellent for digestion and refreshing teas.

How to Grow:

- Thrives in pots (to prevent spreading) or partial shade.
- Likes moist soil but needs good drainage.

Harvesting: Snip leaves regularly to encourage growth.

3. Lavender (Lavandula angustifolia)

Why Grow It: Lavender's calming aroma is perfect for sleep remedies, skin soothers, and natural insect repellents.

How to Grow:

- Needs full sun and well-drained soil.
- Ideal for pots, as it thrives with minimal watering.

Harvesting: Harvest flower stalks before the buds fully open for maximum fragrance and potency.

4. Calendula (Calendula officinalis)

Why Grow It: This bright flower has anti-inflammatory and skin-healing properties.

How to Grow:

- Tolerates a wide range of soils but prefers full sun.
- Self-seeds easily, making it perfect for garden beds.

Harvesting: Collect flowers when fully open and dry them for oils, salves, or teas.

5. Basil (Ocimum basilicum)

Why Grow It: Beyond its culinary uses, basil is excellent for digestion and reducing stress.

How to Grow:

- Thrives in pots with rich, moist soil and full sun.
- Pinch off flowers to keep the plant producing leaves.

Harvesting: Harvest leaves as needed, ideally before the plant flowers.

6. Lemon Balm (Melissa officinalis)

Why Grow It: Known for calming the nervous system and uplifting the mood.

How to Grow:

- Easy to grow in pots or garden beds with partial shade.
- Prefers well-drained soil.

Harvesting: Pick leaves regularly to encourage new growth.

Gardening Tips: Soil, Sunlight, and Seasonal Planting

Growing medicinal herbs successfully depends on understanding the basic needs of your plants. Here's a guide to setting them up for success:

1. Soil

Healthy soil is the foundation of any thriving garden.

- **Well-Drained Soil**: Most herbs, like lavender and chamomile, prefer soil that doesn't retain water. Add sand or perlite to improve drainage for potted plants.
- **Enriched Soil**: For plants like basil or lemon balm, enrich the soil with compost or organic fertilizer for better growth.
- **Testing Soil**: Test your soil's pH with a simple kit. Most herbs thrive in slightly acidic to neutral soil (pH 6–7).

2. Sunlight

Herbs generally love sunlight, but the amount varies depending on the plant.

- **Full Sun (6–8 Hours Daily)**: Lavender, chamomile, and basil thrive in sunny spots.
- **Partial Shade (4–6 Hours Daily)**: Mint, lemon balm, and parsley grow well in shadier areas.
- **Indoor Gardening**: If growing indoors, place herbs near a south-facing window or use grow lights to supplement natural light.

3. Seasonal Planting

Timing is everything when it comes to planting herbs.

- **Cool-Season Herbs**: Start growing chamomile, parsley, and mint in early spring or late summer, as they prefer cooler temperatures.
- **Warm-Season Herbs**: Basil, lavender, and calendula thrive in late spring and summer when the weather is warm.

- **Succession Planting**: Plant herbs in stages to ensure continuous harvests throughout the growing season.

Companion Planting and Natural Pest Control

A healthy apothecary garden relies on balance, where plants help protect one another and pests are controlled naturally.

1. Companion Planting

Pair herbs that support each other's growth and protect against pests.

- **Lavender + Chamomile**: Lavender repels aphids and other pests, protecting chamomile.
- **Basil + Tomatoes**: Basil improves the flavor of tomatoes and deters whiteflies.
- **Mint + Cabbage**: Mint wards off cabbage moths and other insects.

Companion planting also maximizes space, making it perfect for small gardens or pots.

2. Natural Pest Control

Instead of chemical pesticides, use natural methods to protect your garden.

- **Herbal Sprays**: Create a natural pest repellent by mixing garlic, cayenne pepper, and water. Spray directly on plants.
- **Encourage Beneficial Insects**: Attract pollinators like bees and pest-eating insects like ladybugs by planting flowers like calendula or marigolds.
- **Mulching**: Use mulch to suppress weeds, retain moisture, and protect plants from pests like slugs.

Designing Your Apothecary Garden

The layout of your garden should reflect both your space and your needs.

1. Windowsill Apothecary

Perfect For: Small apartments or limited spaces.

Setup: Line up small pots of mint, basil, and parsley along a sunny window. Rotate regularly for even sunlight exposure.

2. Patio or Balcony Garden

Perfect For: Medium spaces with outdoor access.

Setup: Use vertical planters or tiered shelves to grow multiple herbs in a small footprint. Pair tall herbs like lavender with trailing ones like mint for variety.

3. Raised Beds or Garden Plots

Perfect For: Those with yard space who want a more robust apothecary.

Setup: Create a designated herb bed with sections for calming herbs (chamomile, lemon balm), digestive aids (peppermint, fennel), and skincare herbs (calendula, aloe vera).

Growing your own apothecary garden is one of the most fulfilling ways to deepen your relationship with herbal healing. Whether you're tending to a single pot of mint or a sprawling herb bed, every plant you grow becomes a part of your journey toward self-reliance and natural wellness.

2.4 Mastering the Core Techniques

Herbal remedies come in many forms, each tailored to extract the best from your plants and address specific needs. From soothing teas to potent tinctures, and from nourishing salves to effective poultices, learning these core techniques is an essential step in your herbal journey. The good news? These methods are simple, versatile, and deeply rewarding once you understand the basics.

In this chapter, we'll dive into how to make some of the most foundational herbal preparations with step-by-step instructions. By the end, you'll feel confident crafting remedies for yourself and your loved ones.

How to Make Teas, Infusions, and Decoctions

1. Herbal Teas

Teas are the simplest and most widely used herbal preparation, perfect for gentle, daily healing.

What They're Best For:

- Soothing stress (e.g., chamomile tea).
- Digestive discomfort (e.g., peppermint tea).

How to Make an Herbal Tea:

1. Boil 1 cup (8 oz) of water.
2. Add 1 teaspoon of dried herbs (or 2 teaspoons of fresh herbs) to a tea strainer or directly into a cup.
3. Pour the hot water over the herbs.
4. Cover the cup with a lid or plate to trap the steam and steep for 5–10 minutes.
5. Strain, if needed, and enjoy.

Pro Tip: Add honey, lemon, or spices like cinnamon to enhance flavor and benefits.

2. Infusions

Infusions are essentially stronger teas, made to extract more nutrients and medicinal compounds from the herbs.

What They're Best For:

- Nourishing the body with vitamins and minerals (e.g., nettle or oat straw infusions).

- Deep relaxation (e.g., lemon balm infusion).

How to Make an Infusion:

1. Place 1–2 tablespoons of dried herbs in a large jar or teapot.
2. Add 2–3 cups of boiling water.
3. Cover and steep for at least 20 minutes (or up to 8 hours for nutrient-dense herbs like nettle).
4. Strain the liquid and drink warm or cold.

Pro Tip: Store leftover infusion in the refrigerator for up to 24 hours.

3. Decoctions

Decoctions are used for tougher plant materials, like roots, bark, and seeds, which require longer cooking to release their properties.

What They're Best For:

- Supporting the immune system (e.g., elderberry decoction).
- Relieving joint pain (e.g., turmeric or ginger decoction).

How to Make a Decoction:

1. Place 1 tablespoon of dried roots, bark, or seeds in a small saucepan.
2. Add 2 cups of water.
3. Bring to a boil, then reduce the heat and simmer gently for 15–30 minutes.
4. Strain and drink warm.

Pro Tip: Combine decoctions with infusions (e.g., a ginger decoction with chamomile infusion) for a layered remedy.

The Art of Creating Tinctures, Syrups, and Oxymels

1. Tinctures

Tinctures are alcohol-based extracts that preserve the potency of herbs for long-term use.

What They're Best For:

- Quick and easy dosing of concentrated herbs (e.g., echinacea tincture for immunity).
- Strong herbs that aren't palatable in tea form.

How to Make a Tincture:

1. Fill a glass jar halfway with dried herbs (or 3/4 full with fresh herbs).
2. Pour vodka, brandy, or grain alcohol over the herbs, covering them completely.
3. Seal the jar and store it in a cool, dark place for 4–6 weeks. Shake the jar daily.
4. Strain the liquid into a clean dropper bottle and label it.

Pro Tip: Use glycerin instead of alcohol to make alcohol-free tinctures, especially for children.

2. Syrups

Herbal syrups combine the benefits of decoctions with the sweetness of honey, making them palatable for both kids and adults.

What They're Best For:

- Treating coughs and colds (e.g., elderberry syrup).
- Soothing sore throats (e.g., ginger-honey syrup).

How to Make a Syrup:

1. Make a decoction (e.g., simmer 1 cup of elderberries in 2 cups of water for 30 minutes).
2. Strain the liquid and return it to the pot.
3. Add 1 cup of honey (or to taste) and stir until dissolved.
4. Pour into a glass jar or bottle and store in the refrigerator for up to 1 month.

Pro Tip: Add spices like cinnamon, cloves, or ginger for extra flavor and benefits.

3. Oxymels

Oxymels are a tangy blend of vinegar, honey, and herbs, perfect for respiratory and digestive support.

What They're Best For:

- Easing congestion (e.g., thyme oxymel).
- Digestive tonics (e.g., peppermint or fennel oxymel).

How to Make an Oxymel:

1. Combine 1 part dried herbs with 3 parts apple cider vinegar in a glass jar.
2. Seal and steep for 2 weeks, shaking daily.
3. Strain and mix the vinegar infusion with an equal part of honey.
4. Store in a glass bottle and use within 3–6 months.

Step-by-Step Instructions for Balms, Salves, Poultices, and Compresses

1. Balms and Salves

These are oil-based remedies thickened with beeswax, perfect for healing dry skin, cuts, and muscle aches.

How to Make a Basic Salve:

1. Infuse 1 cup of dried herbs (e.g., calendula or arnica) in 1 cup of olive oil by gently heating the mixture in a double boiler for 1–2 hours.
2. Strain the infused oil into a clean jar.
3. Melt 1 ounce of beeswax and stir it into the warm oil.
4. Pour into tins or small jars and let cool before sealing.

Pro Tip: Add a few drops of essential oil (like lavender or tea tree) for extra healing properties.

2. Poultices

Poultices involve applying crushed herbs directly to the skin to draw out toxins or soothe inflammation.

How to Make a Poultice:

1. Crush fresh herbs (e.g., plantain or comfrey) with a mortar and pestle.
2. Spread the herb paste onto a clean cloth or gauze.
3. Apply the cloth to the affected area and secure it with a bandage.

Pro Tip: Warm the poultice slightly for deeper penetration, or cool it to reduce swelling.

3. Compresses

Compresses are cloths soaked in herbal infusions or decoctions, applied to the skin for localized relief.

How to Make a Compress:

1. Soak a clean cloth in a warm herbal infusion (e.g., chamomile for calming skin).
2. Wring out the excess liquid and apply the cloth to the affected area.
3. Leave in place for 10–15 minutes.

Pro Tip: Alternate between warm and cool compresses to stimulate circulation and reduce pain.

Crafting Remedies with Confidence

Mastering these core techniques opens the door to endless possibilities in your home apothecary. Whether you're brewing a calming tea, crafting a soothing salve, or bottling a potent tincture, each preparation brings you closer to the wisdom and power of herbal healing.

With these foundational skills, you're now equipped to explore more advanced remedies and customize them for your needs. In the next part of the book, we'll dive into specific remedies for everyday wellness, showing you how to apply these techniques to create a healthier, more natural life.

Part III: 1000+ Remedies for Everyday Wellness

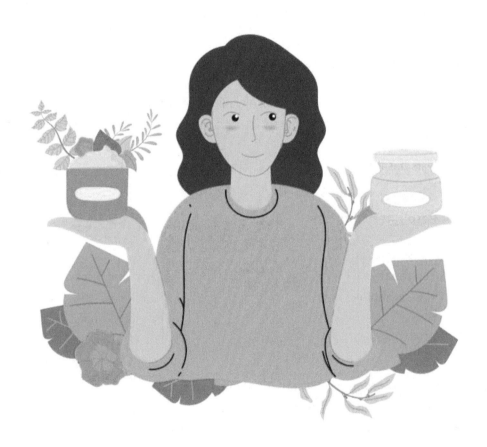

"The remedies we seek are not in far-off laboratories—they are in the soil beneath our feet, the gardens we tend, and the wildflowers that grow unnoticed." - Inspired for this book

Note: Alongside herbal remedies, there are simple daily habits too that complement herbal remedies for a holistic approach to wellness.

3.1 Remedies for Common Ailments

Respiratory Health

1. Ginger and Honey Tea for Cough Relief

- **Ingredients**: 1-inch fresh ginger root (sliced), 1 cup hot water, 1 tsp honey.
- **Method**: Steep ginger slices in hot water for 10 minutes. Strain, add honey, and sip warm.
- **Benefits**: Ginger soothes throat irritation and honey has natural antimicrobial properties.

2. Peppermint Steam Inhalation for Congestion

- **Ingredients**: 2 drops peppermint essential oil, a bowl of hot water.
- **Method**: Add the peppermint oil to hot water. Drape a towel over your head and inhale the steam deeply for 5–10 minutes.
- **Benefits**: Clears nasal passages and relieves sinus congestion.

3. Thyme Tea for Respiratory Infections

- **Ingredients**: 1 tsp dried thyme, 1 cup boiling water.
- **Method**: Steep the thyme in boiling water for 10 minutes. Strain and drink.
- **Benefits**: Thyme is antimicrobial and helps loosen mucus in the lungs.

4. Eucalyptus Chest Rub

- **Ingredients**: 2 tbsp coconut oil, 5 drops eucalyptus essential oil.
- **Method**: Mix the oils and massage into the chest.
- **Benefits**: Eucalyptus opens airways and promotes easier breathing.

5. Elderberry Syrup for Immune Support

- **Ingredients**: 1 cup fresh or dried elderberries, 3 cups water, 1 cup honey.
- **Method**: Simmer elderberries in water for 30 minutes, strain, and mix the liquid with honey. Take 1 tbsp daily.
- **Benefits**: Boosts immunity and shortens the duration of colds and flu.

6. Licorice Root Tea for Sore Throat

- **Ingredients**: 1 tsp licorice root, 1 cup boiling water.
- **Method**: Steep licorice root in boiling water for 10 minutes. Strain and sip warm.
- **Benefits**: Soothes throat inflammation and reduces coughing.

7. Garlic Honey Cough Syrup

- **Ingredients**: 3 cloves garlic (crushed), 1/2 cup raw honey.
- **Method**: Combine garlic and honey in a jar, let it infuse overnight, and take 1 tsp as needed.
- **Benefits**: Garlic fights infections, and honey soothes the throat.

8. Mullein Tea for Clearing Lungs

- **Ingredients**: 1 tsp dried mullein leaves, 1 cup boiling water.
- **Method**: Steep mullein leaves in boiling water for 10 minutes. Strain with a fine mesh to remove tiny hairs and drink.
- **Benefits**: Helps clear mucus and soothe respiratory inflammation.

9. Turmeric Golden Milk for Inflammation

- **Ingredients**: 1 cup milk (dairy or plant-based), 1/2 tsp turmeric powder, 1/4 tsp black pepper, 1 tsp honey.
- **Method**: Warm the milk and whisk in turmeric, black pepper, and honey.
- **Benefits**: Reduces inflammation and supports immune health.

10. Onion and Honey Syrup for Colds

- **Ingredients**: 1 medium onion (sliced), 1/2 cup honey.
- **Method**: Layer onion slices and honey in a jar. Let sit for 6–8 hours, then strain. Take 1 tsp as needed.
- **Benefits**: Onion has expectorant properties, helping to clear mucus.

11. Lemon and Cayenne Gargle for Sore Throats

- **Ingredients**: 1 cup warm water, 1 tbsp lemon juice, 1/4 tsp cayenne pepper.
- **Method**: Mix ingredients and gargle for 30 seconds. Repeat as needed.
- **Benefits**: Lemon cleanses and cayenne reduces throat pain.

12. Marshmallow Root Tea for Dry Cough

- **Ingredients**: 1 tbsp marshmallow root, 1 cup cold water.
- **Method**: Let the root soak in cold water for 4–6 hours, strain, and sip slowly.
- **Benefits**: Soothes irritated mucous membranes and hydrates dry tissues.

13. Pine Needle Infusion for Congestion

- **Ingredients**: 1 tbsp fresh pine needles, 1 cup boiling water.
- **Method**: Steep pine needles in boiling water for 10 minutes. Strain and drink.
- **Benefits**: Clears sinuses and supports respiratory health with its high vitamin C content.

14. Clove Tea for Sore Throats

- **Ingredients**: 3 whole cloves, 1 cup boiling water.
- **Method**: Steep the cloves in boiling water for 10 minutes. Strain and drink.
- **Benefits**: Cloves have anesthetic properties, easing throat pain.

15. Sage Steam for Sinus Relief

- **Ingredients**: 1 tbsp dried sage, a bowl of boiling water.
- **Method**: Add sage to boiling water. Inhale the steam under a towel for 5–10 minutes.
- **Benefits**: Clears sinus congestion and reduces inflammation.

16. Horseradish Tonic for Mucus Clearing

- **Ingredients**: 1 tbsp grated horseradish, 1 tsp apple cider vinegar, 1 tsp honey.
- **Method**: Mix all ingredients and take 1 tsp as needed.
- **Benefits**: Clears nasal passages and loosens mucus.

17. Holy Basil Tea for Respiratory Infections

- **Ingredients**: 1 tsp dried holy basil leaves, 1 cup boiling water.
- **Method**: Steep the leaves in boiling water for 10 minutes. Strain and drink.
- **Benefits**: Reduces respiratory inflammation and supports immunity.

18. Cinnamon and Honey Paste for Coughs

- **Ingredients**: 1 tsp cinnamon powder, 2 tsp honey.
- **Method**: Mix into a paste and take 1 tsp as needed.
- **Benefits**: Cinnamon has warming and antimicrobial properties, while honey soothes the throat.

19. Lavender Steam for Relaxed Breathing

- **Ingredients**: 3 drops lavender essential oil, a bowl of hot water.
- **Method**: Add lavender oil to hot water, inhale deeply for 5–10 minutes.
- **Benefits**: Relaxes airways and reduces stress-related breathing issues.

20. Black Pepper and Honey Tea for Mucus

- **Ingredients**: 1/4 tsp ground black pepper, 1 tsp honey, 1 cup hot water.
- **Method**: Stir the pepper and honey into hot water. Sip slowly.
- **Benefits**: Black pepper breaks up mucus and honey soothes the throat.

Digestive Health

1. Peppermint Tea for Indigestion

- **Ingredients**: 1 tsp dried peppermint leaves, 1 cup boiling water.
- **Method**: Steep peppermint leaves in boiling water for 10 minutes. Strain and sip warm.
- **Benefits**: Relaxes the digestive tract, reducing bloating and gas.

2. Ginger Tea for Nausea

- **Ingredients**: 1-inch fresh ginger root (sliced), 1 cup hot water, honey (optional).
- **Method**: Steep ginger slices in hot water for 10 minutes. Strain and drink warm.
- **Benefits**: Calms nausea and improves digestion by stimulating digestive enzymes.

3. Fennel Seed Tea for Gas

- **Ingredients**: 1 tsp fennel seeds, 1 cup boiling water.
- **Method**: Lightly crush fennel seeds, steep in boiling water for 10 minutes, and strain.
- **Benefits**: Reduces gas and bloating, and supports smoother digestion.

4. Lemon and Warm Water for Morning Detox

- **Ingredients**: Juice of 1/2 lemon, 1 cup warm water.
- **Method**: Squeeze lemon juice into warm water and drink first thing in the morning.
- **Benefits**: Stimulates digestion and detoxifies the liver.

5. Chamomile Tea for Stomach Cramps

- **Ingredients**: 1 tsp dried chamomile flowers, 1 cup boiling water.
- **Method**: Steep chamomile flowers in boiling water for 10 minutes. Strain and drink warm.
- **Benefits**: Soothes the stomach and relieves cramps.

6. Apple Cider Vinegar Tonic for Indigestion

- **Ingredients**: 1 tbsp apple cider vinegar, 1 cup warm water, 1 tsp honey (optional).
- **Method**: Mix vinegar and water, add honey if desired, and drink before meals.
- **Benefits**: Balances stomach acid and aids digestion.

7. Slippery Elm Tea for Heartburn

- **Ingredients**: 1 tsp slippery elm powder, 1 cup warm water.
- **Method**: Mix slippery elm powder into warm water and sip slowly.
- **Benefits**: Coats the stomach lining and reduces acid reflux.

8. Dandelion Root Tea for Liver Support

- **Ingredients**: 1 tsp dried dandelion root, 1 cup boiling water.
- **Method**: Simmer dandelion root in water for 10 minutes, strain, and drink.
- **Benefits**: Supports liver detoxification and improves digestion.

9. Cinnamon Tea for Digestive Warmth

- **Ingredients**: 1 cinnamon stick, 1 cup boiling water.
- **Method**: Steep cinnamon in boiling water for 10 minutes. Strain and sip warm.
- **Benefits**: Relieves gas, bloating, and indigestion.

10. Aloe Vera Juice for Constipation

- **Ingredients**: 2 tbsp fresh aloe vera gel, 1 cup water.
- **Method**: Blend aloe vera gel with water and drink once daily.
- **Benefits**: Promotes regular bowel movements and soothes the gut.

11. Cardamom Tea for Bloating

- **Ingredients**: 4 cardamom pods, 1 cup boiling water.

- **Method**: Crush cardamom pods lightly, steep in boiling water for 10 minutes, and strain.
- **Benefits**: Reduces bloating and supports digestion.

12. Marshmallow Root Infusion for Gut Soothing

- **Ingredients**: 1 tbsp marshmallow root, 1 cup cold water.
- **Method**: Let marshmallow root soak in cold water for 4–6 hours. Strain and sip.
- **Benefits**: Soothes irritated mucous membranes in the gut.

13. Triphala Tonic for Digestive Balance

- **Ingredients**: 1/2 tsp triphala powder, 1 cup warm water.
- **Method**: Mix triphala powder into warm water and drink before bedtime.
- **Benefits**: Balances digestion, supports detoxification, and relieves constipation.

14. Cumin-Coriander-Fennel Tea for Digestion

- **Ingredients**: 1/2 tsp cumin seeds, 1/2 tsp coriander seeds, 1/2 tsp fennel seeds, 2 cups boiling water.
- **Method**: Simmer all seeds in water for 5 minutes, strain, and sip warm.
- **Benefits**: Eases bloating, gas, and sluggish digestion.

15. Licorice Root Tea for Ulcers

- **Ingredients**: 1 tsp licorice root, 1 cup boiling water.
- **Method**: Steep licorice root in boiling water for 10 minutes. Strain and drink.
- **Benefits**: Heals stomach ulcers and soothes inflammation.

16. Mint and Ginger Digestive Water

- **Ingredients**: 1-inch fresh ginger, 5 fresh mint leaves, 4 cups water.
- **Method**: Boil ginger and mint in water for 10 minutes. Strain and refrigerate.
- **Benefits**: Refreshes digestion and relieves bloating.

17. Pineapple and Papaya Smoothie for Digestion

- **Ingredients**: 1/2 cup fresh pineapple, 1/2 cup fresh papaya, 1/2 cup water.
- **Method**: Blend all ingredients until smooth.
- **Benefits**: The natural enzymes (bromelain and papain) break down proteins and ease digestion.

18. Lemon Balm Tea for Digestive Upset

- **Ingredients**: 1 tsp dried lemon balm, 1 cup boiling water.
- **Method**: Steep lemon balm in boiling water for 10 minutes. Strain and drink.
- **Benefits**: Eases nausea and calms an upset stomach.

19. Probiotic Yogurt with Flaxseeds for Gut Health

- **Ingredients**: 1 cup plain probiotic yogurt, 1 tbsp ground flaxseeds.
- **Method**: Mix flaxseeds into yogurt and enjoy.
- **Benefits**: Promotes gut flora balance and regular bowel movements.

20. Turmeric and Black Pepper Tea for Gut Inflammation

- **Ingredients**: 1/2 tsp turmeric powder, 1/4 tsp black pepper, 1 cup warm water.
- **Method**: Stir turmeric and black pepper into warm water and sip.
- **Benefits**: Reduces inflammation and supports gut health.

Pain and Inflammation Relief

1. Turmeric Golden Milk for Inflammation

- **Ingredients**: 1 cup milk (dairy or plant-based), 1/2 tsp turmeric powder, 1/4 tsp black pepper, 1 tsp honey.
- **Method**: Warm the milk and whisk in turmeric, black pepper, and honey. Sip before bedtime.
- **Benefits**: Reduces inflammation and relieves joint and muscle pain.

2. Ginger Tea for Muscle Pain

- **Ingredients**: 1-inch fresh ginger root (sliced), 1 cup boiling water, honey (optional).
- **Method**: Steep ginger in boiling water for 10 minutes, strain, and drink.
- **Benefits**: Ginger's anti-inflammatory compounds help soothe muscle pain and cramps.

3. Arnica Oil for Bruises and Sore Muscles

- **Ingredients**: Arnica-infused oil (store-bought or homemade).
- **Method**: Massage a small amount onto bruised or sore areas twice daily.
- **Benefits**: Reduces swelling, improves circulation, and relieves pain.

4. Willow Bark Tea for Joint Pain

- **Ingredients**: 1 tsp dried willow bark, 1 cup boiling water.
- **Method**: Simmer the bark in boiling water for 10 minutes, strain, and drink.
- **Benefits**: Acts as a natural pain reliever due to its salicin content, similar to aspirin.

5. Epsom Salt Bath for Sore Muscles

- **Ingredients**: 1 cup Epsom salt, warm bathwater.
- **Method**: Dissolve Epsom salt in warm water and soak for 20 minutes.
- **Benefits**: Magnesium in the salt relaxes muscles and reduces inflammation.

6. Lavender Essential Oil for Headaches

- **Ingredients**: 2–3 drops lavender essential oil, carrier oil (e.g., coconut oil).
- **Method**: Dilute lavender oil with a carrier oil and massage into temples or inhale the scent.
- **Benefits**: Calms the mind and relieves tension headaches.

7. Rosemary Infused Oil for Muscle Stiffness

- **Ingredients**: 1/2 cup olive oil, 2 tbsp dried rosemary.
- **Method**: Gently warm the oil with rosemary and let it infuse for 1 hour. Strain and massage into sore areas.
- **Benefits**: Increases circulation and reduces stiffness in muscles and joints.

8. Clove Oil for Toothache Relief

- **Ingredients**: 1 drop clove essential oil, 1/4 tsp carrier oil (like olive oil).
- **Method**: Mix oils, dip a cotton swab into the mixture, and apply to the affected tooth.
- **Benefits**: Clove oil acts as a natural anesthetic and reduces inflammation.

9. Chamomile Compress for Menstrual Cramps

- **Ingredients**: 1 cup chamomile tea (strongly brewed), clean cloth.
- **Method**: Soak the cloth in warm chamomile tea, wring out excess liquid, and place it over the lower abdomen.
- **Benefits**: Relaxes muscles and eases menstrual pain.

10. Cayenne Salve for Joint Pain

- **Ingredients**: 1/4 cup coconut oil, 1 tbsp beeswax, 1 tsp cayenne powder.
- **Method**: Melt the coconut oil and beeswax, stir in cayenne powder, and pour into a jar. Apply sparingly to sore joints.
- **Benefits**: Capsaicin in cayenne reduces pain signals in the nerves.

11. Peppermint Oil for Tension Headaches

- **Ingredients**: 2 drops peppermint essential oil, carrier oil (e.g., almond oil).
- **Method**: Dilute peppermint oil and massage onto temples or the back of the neck.
- **Benefits**: Provides a cooling sensation that relieves headache tension.

12. Dandelion Root Tea for Joint Health

- **Ingredients**: 1 tsp dried dandelion root, 1 cup boiling water.
- **Method**: Simmer dandelion root in boiling water for 10 minutes, strain, and drink.
- **Benefits**: Reduces joint inflammation and supports detoxification.

13. Calendula Salve for Skin Inflammation

- **Ingredients**: 1/2 cup calendula-infused oil, 1 tbsp beeswax.
- **Method**: Melt beeswax, stir into the oil, and pour into a jar. Apply to inflamed skin.
- **Benefits**: Reduces redness, irritation, and swelling.

14. Holy Basil Tea for Stress-Related Pain

- **Ingredients**: 1 tsp dried holy basil leaves, 1 cup boiling water.
- **Method**: Steep holy basil leaves in boiling water for 10 minutes. Strain and drink.
- **Benefits**: Reduces stress-induced muscle tension and inflammation.

15. Ginger and Turmeric Paste for Inflammatory Pain

- **Ingredients**: 1 tsp grated ginger, 1 tsp turmeric powder, 1 tsp honey.
- **Method**: Mix into a paste and take daily with warm water.
- **Benefits**: Combines two powerful anti-inflammatory ingredients for joint and muscle pain.

16. Ice and Peppermint Compress for Migraines

- **Ingredients**: Ice cubes, a few drops of peppermint essential oil, a cloth.

- **Method**: Add peppermint oil to the cloth, wrap ice cubes inside, and apply to the back of the neck.
- **Benefits**: Reduces migraine intensity with cooling and soothing properties.

17. Comfrey Poultice for Sprains

- **Ingredients**: Fresh or dried comfrey leaves, water, clean cloth.
- **Method**: Crush comfrey leaves into a paste, spread on a cloth, and wrap around the injured area.
- **Benefits**: Accelerates healing and reduces pain and swelling in sprains.

18. Black Pepper and Castor Oil Rub for Stiff Joints

- **Ingredients**: 1/4 tsp black pepper, 1 tbsp castor oil.
- **Method**: Warm the oil, mix in black pepper, and massage onto stiff joints.
- **Benefits**: Improves circulation and reduces stiffness and pain.

19. Mustard Seed Bath for Muscle Recovery

- **Ingredients**: 2 tbsp ground mustard seeds, warm bathwater.
- **Method**: Add ground mustard seeds to the bath and soak for 20 minutes.
- **Benefits**: Relieves muscle aches and improves circulation.

20. Aloe Vera Gel for Burn Pain Relief

- **Ingredients**: Fresh aloe vera gel.
- **Method**: Apply a generous amount of aloe vera gel directly to the burn.
- **Benefits**: Soothes pain and reduces inflammation from burns.

Fever and Seasonal Illnesses

1. Yarrow Tea for Fever Reduction

- **Ingredients**: 1 tsp dried yarrow flowers, 1 cup boiling water.
- **Method**: Steep yarrow in boiling water for 10 minutes. Strain and drink warm.
- **Benefits**: Promotes sweating to help break a fever naturally.

2. Elderflower and Peppermint Tea for Flu

- **Ingredients**: 1 tsp elderflowers, 1 tsp peppermint leaves, 1 cup boiling water.

- **Method**: Steep herbs in boiling water for 10 minutes. Strain and sip slowly.
- **Benefits**: Reduces fever, clears congestion, and soothes flu symptoms.

3. Garlic and Honey Immune Booster

- **Ingredients**: 3 crushed garlic cloves, 1/2 cup honey.
- **Method**: Combine garlic and honey in a jar and let infuse for 6–8 hours. Take 1 tsp as needed.
- **Benefits**: Antiviral and immune-boosting properties help fight colds and flu.

4. Lemon, Honey, and Ginger Tea for Colds

- **Ingredients**: Juice of 1/2 lemon, 1-inch fresh ginger (sliced), 1 tsp honey, 1 cup hot water.
- **Method**: Steep ginger in hot water for 10 minutes, then add lemon juice and honey.
- **Benefits**: Reduces congestion, soothes sore throats, and supports the immune system.

5. Cinnamon Tea for Chills

- **Ingredients**: 1 cinnamon stick, 1 cup boiling water.
- **Method**: Steep cinnamon in boiling water for 10 minutes. Strain and drink warm.
- **Benefits**: Warms the body and helps alleviate chills.

6. Onion and Honey Cough Syrup

- **Ingredients**: 1 medium onion (sliced), 1/2 cup honey.
- **Method**: Layer onion slices and honey in a jar. Let sit for 6 hours, strain, and take 1 tsp as needed.
- **Benefits**: Soothes coughs and relieves respiratory congestion.

7. Peppermint Steam for Nasal Congestion

- **Ingredients**: 3 drops peppermint essential oil, a bowl of hot water.
- **Method**: Add peppermint oil to the water, cover your head with a towel, and inhale deeply for 5–10 minutes.
- **Benefits**: Clears sinuses and opens airways.

8. Herbal Fever Bath with Epsom Salt

- **Ingredients**: 1 cup Epsom salt, 1/4 cup dried lavender, chamomile, or rosemary.
- **Method**: Add Epsom salt and herbs to warm bathwater and soak for 20 minutes.
- **Benefits**: Relieves body aches and promotes relaxation.

9. Basil Tea for Mild Fevers

- **Ingredients**: 1 tsp dried basil leaves, 1 cup boiling water.
- **Method**: Steep basil leaves in boiling water for 10 minutes. Strain and drink.
- **Benefits**: Reduces mild fevers and supports recovery.

10. Thyme Tea for Respiratory Infections

- **Ingredients**: 1 tsp dried thyme, 1 cup boiling water.
- **Method**: Steep thyme in boiling water for 10 minutes. Strain and sip slowly.
- **Benefits**: Antimicrobial properties help fight respiratory infections.

11. Cold Compress with Lavender Oil for Fever

- **Ingredients**: A bowl of cool water, 3 drops lavender essential oil, a clean cloth.
- **Method**: Add lavender oil to cool water. Soak the cloth, wring it out, and place it on the forehead.
- **Benefits**: Reduces fever and provides calming relief.

12. Ginger Foot Bath for Fevers

- **Ingredients**: 1-inch fresh ginger (grated), a basin of warm water.
- **Method**: Add grated ginger to warm water and soak feet for 15–20 minutes.
- **Benefits**: Encourages sweating to lower fever and improve circulation.

13. Chamomile and Lemon Balm Tea for Rest

- **Ingredients**: 1 tsp dried chamomile flowers, 1 tsp dried lemon balm leaves, 1 cup boiling water.
- **Method**: Steep herbs in boiling water for 10 minutes. Strain and drink before bed.
- **Benefits**: Promotes restful sleep and relaxation during illness.

14. Spiced Turmeric Tea for Immune Support

- **Ingredients**: 1/2 tsp turmeric powder, 1/4 tsp cinnamon, 1 cup boiling water, honey (optional).
- **Method**: Mix turmeric and cinnamon into boiling water, stir in honey, and sip.
- **Benefits**: Anti-inflammatory and immune-boosting properties support faster recovery.

15. Sage Gargle for Sore Throats

- **Ingredients**: 1 tsp dried sage, 1 cup boiling water, 1/4 tsp salt.

- **Method**: Steep sage in boiling water for 10 minutes, add salt, and gargle.
- **Benefits**: Reduces throat inflammation and kills bacteria.

16. Nettle Tea for Seasonal Allergies

- **Ingredients**: 1 tsp dried nettle leaves, 1 cup boiling water.
- **Method**: Steep nettle in boiling water for 10 minutes. Strain and drink warm.
- **Benefits**: Reduces inflammation and relieves allergy symptoms.

17. Garlic Soup for Immune Boosting

- **Ingredients**: 4 garlic cloves (minced), 1 tbsp olive oil, 2 cups vegetable broth.
- **Method**: Sauté garlic in olive oil, add broth, simmer for 10 minutes, and drink warm.
- **Benefits**: Strengthens the immune system and supports faster recovery.

18. Apple Cider Vinegar Tonic for Fever

- **Ingredients**: 1 tbsp apple cider vinegar, 1 cup warm water, 1 tsp honey.
- **Method**: Mix vinegar and honey into warm water and sip.
- **Benefits**: Helps regulate body temperature and reduce fever.

19. Pine Needle Tea for Vitamin C

- **Ingredients**: 1 tbsp fresh pine needles, 1 cup boiling water.
- **Method**: Steep pine needles in boiling water for 10 minutes, strain, and drink.
- **Benefits**: Boosts immunity and helps combat colds and flu.

20. Warm Compress with Ginger for Aches

- **Ingredients**: 2 tbsp grated ginger, 1 quart hot water, a clean cloth.
- **Method**: Add grated ginger to hot water, soak the cloth, wring it out, and apply to achy areas.
- **Benefits**: Relieves body aches and promotes circulation.

3.2 Remedies for Skin, Hair, and Beauty Care

Skin Healing

1. Witch Hazel Toner for Cuts and Scrapes

- **Ingredients**: 1 tsp witch hazel extract, a cotton ball.
- **Method**: Dab witch hazel onto cuts and scrapes to clean and soothe.
- **Benefits**: Antiseptic and anti-inflammatory properties promote faster healing.

2. Cucumber and Aloe Mask for Sunburn Relief

- **Ingredients**: 1/2 cucumber (blended), 1 tbsp aloe vera gel.
- **Method**: Mix cucumber and aloe, apply to the affected area, and rinse after 20 minutes.
- **Benefits**: Cools the skin, reduces redness, and hydrates sun-damaged skin.

3. Oatmeal Bath for Itchy Skin

- **Ingredients**: 1 cup finely ground oats.
- **Method**: Add oats to a warm bath and soak for 20 minutes.
- **Benefits**: Soothes eczema, rashes, and dry, itchy skin.

4. Lavender Oil Spray for Minor Cuts

- **Ingredients**: 1/4 cup distilled water, 5 drops lavender essential oil.
- **Method**: Mix in a spray bottle and spritz on minor cuts or abrasions.
- **Benefits**: Antiseptic and soothing for minor wounds.

5. Potato Slice for Burns

- **Ingredients**: A fresh potato slice.
- **Method**: Place a raw potato slice directly on the burn for 10–15 minutes.
- **Benefits**: Reduces pain, cools the burn, and prevents blistering.

6. Coconut Oil and Beeswax Lip Balm for Cracked Lips

- **Ingredients**: 2 tbsp coconut oil, 1 tbsp beeswax.
- **Method**: Melt and mix the ingredients, pour into a small tin, and let cool. Apply as needed.
- **Benefits**: Heals cracked, dry lips and locks in moisture.

7. Banana Peel for Bruises

- **Ingredients**: Fresh banana peel.
- **Method**: Place the inside of the banana peel over the bruise for 15 minutes.
- **Benefits**: Reduces swelling and speeds up the fading of bruises.

8. Marshmallow Root Salve for Dry, Cracked Skin

- **Ingredients**: 1/2 cup marshmallow root-infused oil, 1 tbsp beeswax.
- **Method**: Melt beeswax, mix with infused oil, and pour into a jar. Apply to cracked skin.
- **Benefits**: Hydrates and soothes dry, chapped skin.

9. Baking Soda Paste for Poison Ivy

- **Ingredients**: 1 tbsp baking soda, 1 tsp water.
- **Method**: Mix into a paste and apply to poison ivy rash. Rinse after 20 minutes.
- **Benefits**: Neutralizes itchiness and dries out blisters.

10. Turmeric and Yogurt Mask for Scars

- **Ingredients**: 1 tsp turmeric, 2 tbsp plain yogurt.
- **Method**: Mix and apply to scars or dark spots. Rinse off after 15 minutes.
- **Benefits**: Reduces pigmentation and promotes even skin tone.

11. Rosewater and Glycerin Spray for Sensitive Skin

- **Ingredients**: 1/2 cup rosewater, 1 tbsp glycerin.
- **Method**: Combine in a spray bottle and spritz onto irritated skin.
- **Benefits**: Hydrates and soothes redness and sensitivity.

12. Parsley and Honey Poultice for Insect Stings

- **Ingredients**: 1 tbsp fresh parsley (crushed), 1 tsp honey.
- **Method**: Mix into a paste, apply to stings, and cover with a bandage.

- **Benefits**: Reduces swelling and inflammation from stings.

13. Neem Oil for Acne Scars

- **Ingredients**: 2 drops neem oil, 1 tsp carrier oil (e.g., almond oil).
- **Method**: Mix oils and apply to acne scars nightly.
- **Benefits**: Antibacterial and scar-fading properties promote clear skin.

14. Calendula Ice Cubes for Irritated Skin

- **Ingredients**: 1 cup calendula tea, ice cube tray.
- **Method**: Brew calendula tea, pour into ice trays, and freeze. Rub cubes on irritated skin.
- **Benefits**: Reduces inflammation and cools itchy, red areas.

15. Carrot Paste for Skin Repair

- **Ingredients**: 1 carrot (boiled and mashed), 1 tsp honey.
- **Method**: Mix into a paste and apply to damaged skin. Rinse after 20 minutes.
- **Benefits**: Rich in beta-carotene, helps repair and nourish damaged skin.

16. Flaxseed Gel for Dry Skin

- **Ingredients**: 2 tbsp flaxseeds, 1 cup water.
- **Method**: Simmer flaxseeds in water until gel forms. Strain and apply to dry patches.
- **Benefits**: Locks in moisture and soothes irritation.

17. Comfrey Leaf Compress for Wounds

- **Ingredients**: Fresh comfrey leaves, boiling water.
- **Method**: Soak leaves in boiling water, let cool slightly, and apply as a compress to wounds.
- **Benefits**: Speeds wound healing and reduces inflammation.

18. Milk and Rice Flour Scrub for Exfoliation

- **Ingredients**: 1 tbsp rice flour, 2 tbsp milk.
- **Method**: Mix into a paste, gently massage onto the skin, and rinse.
- **Benefits**: Removes dead skin cells and brightens dull skin.

19. Papaya and Honey Mask for Skin Regeneration

- **Ingredients**: 2 tbsp mashed papaya, 1 tsp honey.
- **Method**: Mix and apply to the skin. Leave on for 15 minutes and rinse.
- **Benefits**: Papaya enzymes promote skin regeneration and reduce scars.

20. Beetroot Juice for Skin Brightening

- **Ingredients**: Fresh beetroot juice (diluted).
- **Method**: Dab onto the skin with a cotton pad and rinse after 10 minutes.
- **Benefits**: Improves skin tone and reduces dullness.

21. Tea Tree Oil Spot Treatment for Pimples

- **Ingredients**: 1 drop tea tree oil, 1 tsp carrier oil.
- **Method**: Mix and dab onto pimples with a cotton swab.
- **Benefits**: Antibacterial properties help dry out and heal pimples.

22. Sea Salt Scrub for Rough Skin

- **Ingredients**: 1/2 cup sea salt, 1/4 cup olive oil.
- **Method**: Mix and gently scrub onto rough areas like elbows and knees.
- **Benefits**: Exfoliates and softens rough patches.

23. Coconut Milk and Oatmeal Face Wash

- **Ingredients**: 2 tbsp oatmeal, 3 tbsp coconut milk.
- **Method**: Mix into a paste, gently massage onto the face, and rinse.
- **Benefits**: Cleanses, moisturizes, and soothes sensitive skin.

24. Apple Cider Vinegar Rinse for Itchy Scalp

- **Ingredients**: 1/4 cup apple cider vinegar, 1/2 cup water.
- **Method**: Mix and pour over the scalp after shampooing.
- **Benefits**: Reduces scalp irritation and promotes healing.

25. Clay and Rosewater Mask for Detoxing Skin

- **Ingredients**: 1 tbsp bentonite clay, 2 tbsp rosewater.
- **Method**: Mix into a paste, apply to the face, and rinse after 15 minutes.
- **Benefits**: Draws out impurities and detoxifies the skin.

Everyday Skincare

1. Rosewater Toner for Hydration

- **Ingredients**: 1/2 cup rosewater, 1 tsp glycerin (optional).
- **Method**: Combine and store in a spray bottle. Use as a toner after cleansing.
- **Benefits**: Hydrates and balances the skin's pH.

2. Milk Cleanser for Soft Skin

- **Ingredients**: 2 tbsp raw milk, a cotton pad.
- **Method**: Dab milk onto the skin with the cotton pad, leave for 5 minutes, and rinse.
- **Benefits**: Gently cleanses and nourishes the skin.

3. Green Tea Ice Cubes for Morning Glow

- **Ingredients**: 1 cup green tea, ice cube tray.
- **Method**: Brew green tea, pour into the tray, and freeze. Rub an ice cube on your face in the morning.
- **Benefits**: Reduces puffiness, tightens pores, and refreshes skin.

4. Cucumber and Honey Gel for Hydration

- **Ingredients**: 2 tbsp cucumber juice, 1 tsp honey.
- **Method**: Mix and apply to the skin. Leave for 15 minutes and rinse.
- **Benefits**: Hydrates and soothes tired, dry skin.

5. Almond and Oat Exfoliator for Gentle Scrubbing

- **Ingredients**: 2 tbsp ground almonds, 1 tbsp oatmeal, 1 tbsp water.
- **Method**: Mix into a paste, gently scrub the skin, and rinse.
- **Benefits**: Exfoliates dead skin cells and smooths the complexion.

6. Aloe Vera and Lemon Brightening Mask

- **Ingredients**: 2 tbsp aloe vera gel, 1 tsp fresh lemon juice.
- **Method**: Mix and apply to the face. Rinse after 10 minutes.
- **Benefits**: Brightens the skin and reduces dark spots.

7. Yogurt and Honey Cleanser

- **Ingredients**: 1 tbsp plain yogurt, 1 tsp honey.
- **Method**: Mix and massage onto the skin. Leave for 5 minutes, then rinse.
- **Benefits**: Cleanses while moisturizing and softening the skin.

8. Avocado Moisturizing Mask

- **Ingredients**: 1/2 ripe avocado, 1 tsp olive oil.
- **Method**: Mash avocado, mix with olive oil, and apply to the face. Leave for 15 minutes and rinse.
- **Benefits**: Deeply hydrates and nourishes dry skin.

9. Witch Hazel and Tea Tree Spot Treatment

- **Ingredients**: 1 tsp witch hazel, 2 drops tea tree oil.
- **Method**: Mix and apply to blemishes with a cotton swab.
- **Benefits**: Clears acne and reduces inflammation.

10. Banana and Sugar Lip Scrub

- **Ingredients**: 1 tsp mashed banana, 1 tsp sugar.
- **Method**: Mix and gently scrub your lips. Rinse and follow with a lip balm.
- **Benefits**: Exfoliates and softens dry lips.

11. Jojoba Oil Moisturizer for Oily Skin

- **Ingredients**: 3–4 drops jojoba oil.
- **Method**: Massage into freshly cleansed skin.
- **Benefits**: Balances oil production without clogging pores.

12. Coffee Grounds Scrub for Radiance

- **Ingredients**: 2 tbsp used coffee grounds, 1 tbsp coconut oil.
- **Method**: Mix and gently massage onto damp skin. Rinse thoroughly.
- **Benefits**: Exfoliates and improves circulation, leaving skin radiant.

13. Mint and Basil Face Mist for Freshness

- **Ingredients**: 1/2 cup mint tea, 1/4 cup basil tea, spray bottle.
- **Method**: Mix the teas, pour into the bottle, and spritz on the face throughout the day.

- **Benefits**: Refreshes and revitalizes tired skin.

14. Rosehip Oil Serum for Anti-Aging

- **Ingredients**: 2–3 drops rosehip oil.
- **Method**: Warm the oil in your palms and press gently into the skin after cleansing.
- **Benefits**: Reduces fine lines and improves skin elasticity.

15. Coconut Milk Toner for Smooth Skin

- **Ingredients**: 2 tbsp coconut milk, a cotton pad.
- **Method**: Dab the coconut milk onto the skin and rinse after 5 minutes.
- **Benefits**: Softens skin and provides natural hydration.

16. Rice Water Rinse for Clear Skin

- **Ingredients**: 1/2 cup rice water (leftover from rinsing uncooked rice).
- **Method**: Use rice water to rinse your face, then pat dry.
- **Benefits**: Tightens pores and brightens the skin.

17. Papaya Enzyme Mask for Dead Skin

- **Ingredients**: 2 tbsp mashed papaya.
- **Method**: Apply directly to the skin, leave for 10 minutes, and rinse.
- **Benefits**: Gently removes dead skin cells and promotes regeneration.

18. Raw Honey Spot Treatment for Dry Patches

- **Ingredients**: 1 tsp raw honey.
- **Method**: Dab honey directly onto dry patches and leave for 10 minutes. Rinse with warm water.
- **Benefits**: Deeply moisturizes and heals dry skin.

19. Chamomile and Oat Face Mask for Sensitive Skin

- **Ingredients**: 2 tbsp oatmeal, 1 tbsp chamomile tea.
- **Method**: Mix into a paste, apply to the face, and rinse after 15 minutes.
- **Benefits**: Calms redness and soothes irritation.

20. Tomato Pulp Mask for Oily Skin

- **Ingredients**: 1/2 ripe tomato (blended).
- **Method**: Apply tomato pulp to the skin, leave for 10 minutes, and rinse.
- **Benefits**: Reduces excess oil and tightens pores.

21. Almond Oil Eye Cream for Dark Circles

- **Ingredients**: 1 tsp almond oil.
- **Method**: Gently massage almond oil under your eyes before bed.
- **Benefits**: Reduces puffiness and lightens dark circles.

22. Cucumber and Mint Toner for Cooling

- **Ingredients**: 1/4 cucumber (blended), 2 tbsp mint tea.
- **Method**: Mix and store in a spray bottle. Use as a cooling toner.
- **Benefits**: Calms irritation and cools the skin.

23. Apple Cider Vinegar Toner for Acne-Prone Skin

- **Ingredients**: 1 tbsp apple cider vinegar, 2 tbsp water.
- **Method**: Mix and apply with a cotton pad after cleansing.
- **Benefits**: Reduces acne and balances the skin's pH.

24. Shea Butter Moisturizer for Dry Skin

- **Ingredients**: 1 tsp raw shea butter.
- **Method**: Warm in your palms and massage into dry areas.
- **Benefits**: Locks in moisture and soothes flaky skin.

25. Lemon Sugar Scrub for Bright Skin

- **Ingredients**: 1 tbsp sugar, 1 tsp fresh lemon juice.
- **Method**: Mix and gently scrub onto damp skin. Rinse thoroughly.
- **Benefits**: Exfoliates and brightens dull skin.

Hair Care

1. Aloe Vera Hair Mask for Dry Hair

- **Ingredients**: 2 tbsp aloe vera gel, 1 tbsp coconut oil.
- **Method**: Mix and apply to your scalp and hair. Leave for 30 minutes and rinse.
- **Benefits**: Deeply hydrates and soothes dry, frizzy hair.

2. Apple Cider Vinegar Rinse for Dandruff

- **Ingredients**: 2 tbsp apple cider vinegar, 1 cup water.
- **Method**: Mix and pour over your scalp after shampooing. Let sit for 5 minutes, then rinse.
- **Benefits**: Balances scalp pH and reduces dandruff.

3. Fenugreek Seed Paste for Hair Growth

- **Ingredients**: 2 tbsp fenugreek seeds (soaked overnight), water.
- **Method**: Blend the soaked seeds into a paste, apply to the scalp, and leave for 30 minutes. Rinse thoroughly.
- **Benefits**: Strengthens roots and stimulates hair growth.

4. Onion Juice for Hair Fall

- **Ingredients**: Juice of 1 onion.
- **Method**: Extract onion juice, apply to the scalp, leave for 20 minutes, and rinse with mild shampoo.
- **Benefits**: Boosts circulation and reduces hair fall.

5. Coconut Milk for Nourishment

- **Ingredients**: 1/2 cup coconut milk.
- **Method**: Massage coconut milk into your scalp and hair, leave for 20 minutes, and rinse.
- **Benefits**: Adds shine and strengthens hair strands.

6. Rosemary Hair Rinse for Hair Growth

- **Ingredients**: 2 tbsp dried rosemary, 2 cups boiling water.
- **Method**: Steep rosemary in boiling water, let it cool, and pour over hair as a final rinse.
- **Benefits**: Stimulates hair follicles and promotes growth.

7. Castor Oil Scalp Treatment for Thick Hair

- **Ingredients**: 2 tbsp castor oil, 1 tbsp coconut oil.
- **Method**: Mix oils, warm slightly, and massage into the scalp. Leave overnight and rinse in the morning.
- **Benefits**: Thickens hair and strengthens roots.

8. Egg Yolk Mask for Protein Repair

- **Ingredients**: 1 egg yolk, 1 tbsp olive oil.
- **Method**: Mix and apply to damp hair. Leave for 20 minutes and rinse with cool water.
- **Benefits**: Repairs damage and strengthens weak strands.

9. Hibiscus and Coconut Oil Paste for Shine

- **Ingredients**: 4 fresh hibiscus flowers, 2 tbsp coconut oil.
- **Method**: Blend hibiscus flowers into a paste, mix with coconut oil, and apply to hair. Leave for 30 minutes, then rinse.
- **Benefits**: Restores natural shine and softness.

10. Green Tea Rinse for Hair Fall

- **Ingredients**: 1 cup brewed green tea.
- **Method**: Use cooled green tea as a final rinse after shampooing.
- **Benefits**: Reduces hair fall and strengthens hair follicles.

11. Avocado and Banana Mask for Dry Hair

- **Ingredients**: 1/2 avocado, 1/2 banana, 1 tbsp honey.
- **Method**: Blend into a smooth paste, apply to hair, and rinse after 30 minutes.
- **Benefits**: Deeply nourishes and hydrates dry hair.

12. Lemon Juice Rinse for Oily Hair

- **Ingredients**: Juice of 1 lemon, 1 cup water.
- **Method**: Dilute lemon juice in water and pour over hair. Rinse after 5 minutes.
- **Benefits**: Removes excess oil and adds shine.

13. Yogurt Hair Mask for Dandruff

- **Ingredients**: 1/2 cup plain yogurt, 1 tsp honey.
- **Method**: Apply to the scalp and hair, leave for 20 minutes, and rinse with lukewarm water.
- **Benefits**: Moisturizes the scalp and reduces dandruff.

14. Neem Oil Treatment for Scalp Health

- **Ingredients**: 1 tsp neem oil, 2 tbsp carrier oil (e.g., coconut or olive oil).
- **Method**: Mix oils, apply to the scalp, leave for 30 minutes, and rinse with shampoo.
- **Benefits**: Fights scalp infections and promotes healthy hair growth.

15. Rice Water Rinse for Strengthening

- **Ingredients**: 1 cup rice water (fermented for 24 hours).
- **Method**: Use as a hair rinse after shampooing, leave for 5 minutes, and rinse.
- **Benefits**: Strengthens hair and improves elasticity.

16. Tea Tree and Aloe Scalp Gel for Itching

- **Ingredients**: 2 tbsp aloe vera gel, 2 drops tea tree oil.
- **Method**: Mix and apply to the scalp, leave for 15 minutes, and rinse.
- **Benefits**: Reduces itching and soothes scalp irritation.

17. Bhringraj Oil for Hair Growth

- **Ingredients**: 2 tbsp bhringraj oil.
- **Method**: Warm slightly and massage into the scalp. Leave overnight and rinse.
- **Benefits**: Encourages hair growth and prevents premature graying.

18. Baking Soda Clarifying Rinse

- **Ingredients**: 1 tbsp baking soda, 1 cup water.
- **Method**: Mix and use as a rinse to remove product buildup.
- **Benefits**: Cleanses the scalp and restores shine.

19. Curry Leaves and Coconut Oil Infusion

- **Ingredients**: A handful of curry leaves, 1/2 cup coconut oil.
- **Method**: Heat the curry leaves in coconut oil, cool, strain, and massage into the scalp.
- **Benefits**: Strengthens hair and prevents hair fall.

20. Honey and Olive Oil Conditioner

- **Ingredients**: 2 tbsp honey, 1 tbsp olive oil.
- **Method**: Mix and apply to the hair. Leave for 20 minutes and rinse.
- **Benefits**: Conditions and adds natural shine.

21. Peppermint Oil Scalp Massage for Circulation

- **Ingredients**: 2 drops peppermint oil, 1 tbsp carrier oil (e.g., jojoba oil).
- **Method**: Mix and massage into the scalp for 5 minutes.
- **Benefits**: Improves circulation and stimulates hair follicles.

22. Black Tea Rinse for Darker Hair

- **Ingredients**: 1 cup brewed black tea.
- **Method**: Use as a final rinse after shampooing to enhance natural dark tones.
- **Benefits**: Adds shine and deepens dark hair color.

23. Beer Rinse for Volume

- **Ingredients**: 1/2 cup flat beer.
- **Method**: Pour over clean hair, leave for 5 minutes, and rinse with cool water.
- **Benefits**: Adds volume and luster to fine hair.

24. Flaxseed Gel for Curl Definition

- **Ingredients**: 2 tbsp flaxseeds, 1 cup water.
- **Method**: Simmer flaxseeds in water, strain the gel, and apply to damp hair.
- **Benefits**: Defines curls and reduces frizz.

25. Argan Oil Serum for Frizz Control

- **Ingredients**: 2–3 drops argan oil.
- **Method**: Rub oil between palms and smooth onto the ends of your hair.
- **Benefits**: Tames frizz and adds shine.

Anti-Aging and Glow

1. Rosehip Oil Night Serum

- **Ingredients**: 3 drops rosehip oil, 2 drops jojoba oil.
- **Method**: Mix the oils in your palms and massage gently into your skin before bed.
- **Benefits**: Reduces fine lines and restores skin elasticity overnight.

2. Avocado and Honey Hydrating Mask

- **Ingredients**: 1/4 ripe avocado, 1 tsp raw honey.
- **Method**: Mash the avocado, mix with honey, apply to the face, and rinse after 15 minutes.
- **Benefits**: Deeply moisturizes and plumps the skin for a youthful glow.

3. Pomegranate Seed Scrub for Radiance

- **Ingredients**: 2 tbsp pomegranate seeds (crushed), 1 tsp sugar, 1 tsp olive oil.
- **Method**: Mix and gently massage onto the skin. Rinse thoroughly.
- **Benefits**: Exfoliates dead skin cells and enhances skin's natural glow.

4. Green Tea Ice Facial

- **Ingredients**: 1 cup green tea, ice cube tray.
- **Method**: Brew green tea, freeze in an ice tray, and rub cubes on your face in the morning.
- **Benefits**: Tightens pores and reduces puffiness, leaving skin refreshed.

5. Turmeric and Yogurt Brightening Mask

- **Ingredients**: 1 tsp turmeric powder, 2 tbsp plain yogurt.
- **Method**: Mix and apply to the face. Rinse off after 10–15 minutes.
- **Benefits**: Evens out skin tone and reduces age spots.

6. Argan Oil Eye Treatment

- **Ingredients**: 2 drops argan oil.
- **Method**: Dab oil under the eyes and gently massage before bed.
- **Benefits**: Hydrates and reduces the appearance of fine lines and crow's feet.

7. Carrot and Honey Face Mask for Wrinkles

- **Ingredients**: 1 boiled carrot (mashed), 1 tsp honey.
- **Method**: Mix and apply to the face. Leave for 20 minutes and rinse.
- **Benefits**: Rich in beta-carotene, it smooths wrinkles and rejuvenates the skin.

8. Cucumber and Aloe Vera Gel Mask

- **Ingredients**: 2 tbsp cucumber juice, 1 tbsp aloe vera gel.
- **Method**: Mix and apply to the face. Leave for 15 minutes and rinse.
- **Benefits**: Soothes, hydrates, and promotes glowing skin.

9. Papaya Enzyme Mask for Skin Renewal

- **Ingredients**: 2 tbsp mashed papaya.
- **Method**: Apply directly to the skin, leave for 10 minutes, and rinse.
- **Benefits**: Removes dead skin cells and promotes skin regeneration.

10. Almond Oil and Milk Cleanser

- **Ingredients**: 1 tsp almond oil, 2 tbsp raw milk.
- **Method**: Mix and gently massage into the skin, then rinse.
- **Benefits**: Cleanses and softens skin while reducing dullness.

11. Hibiscus Tea Toner

- **Ingredients**: 1 cup hibiscus tea, spray bottle.
- **Method**: Brew hibiscus tea, cool it, and pour into a spray bottle. Use as a toner.
- **Benefits**: Rich in antioxidants, it firms the skin and enhances glow.

12. Coconut Oil and Coffee Scrub

- **Ingredients**: 2 tbsp coffee grounds, 1 tbsp coconut oil.
- **Method**: Mix and gently scrub onto damp skin. Rinse thoroughly.
- **Benefits**: Stimulates circulation and reduces the appearance of dull skin.

13. Glycerin and Rosewater Glow Serum

- **Ingredients**: 1 tsp glycerin, 2 tbsp rosewater.
- **Method**: Mix and apply a few drops to your face after cleansing.
- **Benefits**: Locks in moisture and provides a dewy glow.

14. Lemon and Olive Oil Anti-Wrinkle Massage

- **Ingredients**: 1 tsp lemon juice, 1 tbsp olive oil.
- **Method**: Mix and gently massage into the skin for 5 minutes. Rinse with warm water.
- **Benefits**: Brightens skin and reduces the appearance of fine lines.

15. Rice Flour and Milk Anti-Aging Mask

- **Ingredients**: 1 tbsp rice flour, 2 tbsp milk.
- **Method**: Mix into a paste, apply to the face, and rinse after 15 minutes.
- **Benefits**: Tightens skin and reduces wrinkles.

16. Flaxseed Gel for Firming

- **Ingredients**: 1 tbsp flaxseeds, 1 cup water.
- **Method**: Simmer flaxseeds in water until gel forms. Apply to the face and rinse after 20 minutes.
- **Benefits**: Firms the skin and enhances elasticity.

17. Beetroot Juice for Rosy Glow

- **Ingredients**: Fresh beetroot juice (diluted).
- **Method**: Dab onto the skin with a cotton pad and rinse after 10 minutes.
- **Benefits**: Improves skin tone and provides a natural blush.

18. Chamomile and Honey Soothing Mask

- **Ingredients**: 1 tbsp chamomile tea, 1 tsp honey.
- **Method**: Mix and apply to the skin. Rinse after 15 minutes.
- **Benefits**: Calms inflammation and brightens dull skin.

19. Neem and Turmeric Anti-Aging Mask

- **Ingredients**: 1 tsp neem powder, 1/2 tsp turmeric, 2 tbsp yogurt.
- **Method**: Mix and apply to the face. Rinse after 15 minutes.
- **Benefits**: Detoxifies the skin and prevents early signs of aging.

20. Grapeseed Oil Massage for Elasticity

- **Ingredients**: 2–3 drops grapeseed oil.

- **Method**: Warm the oil in your palms and gently massage into the skin.
- **Benefits**: Firms skin and reduces fine lines.

21. Turmeric and Sandalwood Brightening Pack

- **Ingredients**: 1 tsp turmeric, 1 tbsp sandalwood powder, water.
- **Method**: Mix into a paste, apply to the face, and rinse after 15 minutes.
- **Benefits**: Brightens the skin and evens out skin tone.

22. Orange Peel Powder Scrub

- **Ingredients**: 1 tbsp orange peel powder, 1 tsp honey.
- **Method**: Mix and gently scrub your face. Rinse thoroughly.
- **Benefits**: Removes dead skin and provides a radiant glow.

23. Shea Butter and Vitamin E Moisturizer

- **Ingredients**: 1 tbsp shea butter, 1 capsule vitamin E oil.
- **Method**: Mix and apply to the face after cleansing.
- **Benefits**: Hydrates and restores elasticity.

24. Egg White and Lemon Tightening Mask

- **Ingredients**: 1 egg white, 1 tsp lemon juice.
- **Method**: Whisk together, apply to the face, and rinse after 10 minutes.
- **Benefits**: Tightens pores and reduces wrinkles.

25. Honey and Cinnamon Glow Mask

- **Ingredients**: 1 tsp honey, 1/4 tsp cinnamon powder.
- **Method**: Mix and apply to the skin. Rinse after 10 minutes.
- **Benefits**: Boosts circulation and leaves skin glowing.

3.3 Stress, Sleep, and Mental Wellness

Relaxation and Anxiety Relief

1. Chamomile Tea for Calmness

- **Ingredients**: 1 tsp dried chamomile flowers, 1 cup boiling water.
- **Method**: Steep chamomile flowers in boiling water for 10 minutes. Strain and sip warm.
- **Benefits**: Calms the nervous system and promotes relaxation.

2. Lemon Balm Tea for Anxiety

- **Ingredients**: 1 tsp dried lemon balm, 1 cup boiling water.
- **Method**: Steep lemon balm in boiling water for 10 minutes. Strain and drink.
- **Benefits**: Relieves stress and soothes anxious thoughts.

3. Lavender Essential Oil Diffusion

- **Ingredients**: 5 drops lavender essential oil, water, a diffuser.
- **Method**: Add oil to a diffuser filled with water and let the aroma fill your space.
- **Benefits**: Reduces stress, promotes relaxation, and helps with sleep.

4. Ashwagandha Latte for Stress Relief

- **Ingredients**: 1/2 tsp ashwagandha powder, 1 cup warm milk, 1 tsp honey.
- **Method**: Mix ashwagandha into the milk, stir in honey, and drink.
- **Benefits**: Balances cortisol levels and supports relaxation.

5. Epsom Salt Bath

- **Ingredients**: 1 cup Epsom salt, warm bathwater.
- **Method**: Dissolve Epsom salt in the bathwater and soak for 20 minutes.
- **Benefits**: Relaxes muscles and calms the mind.

6. Passionflower Tea for Deep Calm

- **Ingredients**: 1 tsp dried passionflower, 1 cup boiling water.

- **Method**: Steep passionflower in boiling water for 10 minutes. Strain and sip.
- **Benefits**: Reduces anxiety and promotes relaxation.

7. Holy Basil Tonic for Stress

- **Ingredients**: 1 tsp dried holy basil leaves, 1 cup boiling water.
- **Method**: Steep basil leaves in boiling water for 10 minutes. Strain and drink.
- **Benefits**: Reduces cortisol and supports emotional balance.

8. Peppermint Steam Inhalation

- **Ingredients**: 2 drops peppermint essential oil, bowl of hot water.
- **Method**: Add peppermint oil to hot water, cover your head with a towel, and inhale deeply.
- **Benefits**: Reduces tension and clears the mind.

9. Lavender and Chamomile Bath Soak

- **Ingredients**: 1/2 cup dried lavender, 1/2 cup dried chamomile, muslin bag, warm bathwater.
- **Method**: Place herbs in a muslin bag and soak in your bath. Relax for 20 minutes.
- **Benefits**: Eases stress and soothes muscles.

10. Warm Milk with Nutmeg for Relaxation

- **Ingredients**: 1 cup warm milk, a pinch of nutmeg.
- **Method**: Stir nutmeg into the milk and drink before bed.
- **Benefits**: Promotes better sleep and calms the mind.

11. Bergamot Roll-On for Anxiety Relief

- **Ingredients**: 2 drops bergamot essential oil, 1 tsp carrier oil.
- **Method**: Mix oils, apply to your wrists or temples, and inhale deeply.
- **Benefits**: Uplifts mood and reduces anxiety.

12. Dark Chocolate for Stress Relief

- **Ingredients**: 1 small piece of dark chocolate (70% or higher).
- **Method**: Slowly savor the chocolate to enjoy its calming effects.
- **Benefits**: Contains magnesium, which reduces stress and boosts mood.

13. Lemon and Honey Anti-Anxiety Drink

- **Ingredients**: Juice of 1/2 lemon, 1 tsp honey, 1 cup warm water.
- **Method**: Mix all ingredients and sip slowly.
- **Benefits**: Hydrates the body and soothes the mind.

14. Ylang-Ylang Massage Oil

- **Ingredients**: 3 drops ylang-ylang oil, 2 tbsp carrier oil.
- **Method**: Mix oils and massage onto the shoulders and neck.
- **Benefits**: Relaxes tense muscles and promotes emotional balance.

15. Rose Petal Tea for Emotional Calm

- **Ingredients**: 1 tsp dried rose petals, 1 cup boiling water.
- **Method**: Steep petals in boiling water for 10 minutes. Strain and drink.
- **Benefits**: Balances emotions and provides a calming effect.

16. Rosemary and Lemon Spray for Focus

- **Ingredients**: 2 drops rosemary oil, 2 drops lemon oil, 1 cup water, spray bottle.
- **Method**: Mix all ingredients in a spray bottle and spritz your space.
- **Benefits**: Clears mental fatigue and improves focus.

17. Green Tea Ice Cubes for Refreshment

- **Ingredients**: 1 cup brewed green tea, ice cube tray.
- **Method**: Freeze green tea in ice trays and rub a cube on your face in the morning.
- **Benefits**: Reduces puffiness and refreshes the skin.

18. Valerian Root Tea for Better Sleep

- **Ingredients**: 1/2 tsp valerian root, 1 cup boiling water.
- **Method**: Steep valerian root in boiling water for 10 minutes. Strain and sip.
- **Benefits**: Relaxes the mind and promotes restful sleep.

19. Lavender Pillow Mist

- **Ingredients**: 1/2 cup water, 5 drops lavender oil, spray bottle.
- **Method**: Mix water and lavender oil in a spray bottle. Spritz onto your pillow before bed.

- **Benefits**: Encourages relaxation and better sleep.

20. Peppermint Foot Soak

- **Ingredients**: 1/4 cup dried peppermint, warm water.
- **Method**: Add peppermint to a basin of warm water and soak feet for 15 minutes.
- **Benefits**: Relaxes tired feet and refreshes the mind.

21. Guided Meditation with Sandalwood Oil

- **Ingredients**: 1 drop sandalwood oil.
- **Method**: Rub oil onto your palms, inhale deeply, and listen to a guided meditation.
- **Benefits**: Grounds the mind and encourages deep relaxation.

22. Holy Basil and Mint Tea

- **Ingredients**: 1/2 tsp dried holy basil, 1/2 tsp dried mint, 1 cup boiling water.
- **Method**: Steep both herbs in boiling water for 10 minutes. Strain and drink.
- **Benefits**: Reduces anxiety and refreshes the mind.

23. Chamomile and Fennel Tea

- **Ingredients**: 1 tsp dried chamomile, 1/2 tsp fennel seeds, 1 cup boiling water.
- **Method**: Steep both in boiling water for 10 minutes. Strain and drink.
- **Benefits**: Eases digestion and calms the body.

24. Flaxseed Gel for Scalp Relaxation

- **Ingredients**: 1 tbsp flaxseeds, 1 cup water.
- **Method**: Simmer flaxseeds in water until a gel forms. Apply to the scalp and rinse after 20 minutes.
- **Benefits**: Soothes the scalp and reduces stress.

25. Honey and Turmeric Tea

- **Ingredients**: 1/2 tsp turmeric powder, 1 tsp honey, 1 cup warm water.
- **Method**: Mix turmeric and honey into warm water and drink.
- **Benefits**: Reduces inflammation and promotes mental calmness.

26. Beetroot Juice for Energy and Calm

- **Ingredients**: 1/2 cup fresh beetroot juice.
- **Method**: Drink chilled beetroot juice slowly.
- **Benefits**: Provides natural energy while calming the mind.

27. Cardamom and Cinnamon Tea

- **Ingredients**: 2 cardamom pods, 1 cinnamon stick, 1 cup boiling water.
- **Method**: Steep spices in boiling water for 10 minutes. Strain and sip.
- **Benefits**: Provides warmth and relieves stress.

28. Almond and Banana Smoothie

- **Ingredients**: 1 banana, 1 cup almond milk, 1 tsp honey.
- **Method**: Blend ingredients into a smoothie and enjoy.
- **Benefits**: Rich in magnesium to calm the body.

29. Aloe and Mint Cooling Gel

- **Ingredients**: 2 tbsp aloe vera gel, 1 tsp crushed mint leaves.
- **Method**: Mix and apply to the skin for 15 minutes. Rinse with cool water.
- **Benefits**: Refreshes and calms the skin.

30. Sandalwood and Rose Massage Blend

- **Ingredients**: 2 drops sandalwood oil, 2 drops rose oil, 1 tbsp carrier oil.
- **Method**: Mix oils and massage onto the temples and neck.
- **Benefits**: Promotes emotional balance and deep relaxation.

Better Sleep

1. Chamomile Tea for Relaxation

- **Ingredients**: 1 tsp dried chamomile flowers, 1 cup boiling water.
- **Method**: Steep chamomile flowers in boiling water for 10 minutes. Strain and sip warm 30 minutes before bed.
- **Benefits**: Calms the nervous system and promotes relaxation.

2. Lavender Pillow Spray

- **Ingredients**: 1/2 cup distilled water, 5 drops lavender essential oil, a spray bottle.
- **Method**: Mix water and oil in the bottle, shake well, and spritz on your pillow before bed.
- **Benefits**: Encourages relaxation and helps with falling asleep.

3. Warm Milk with Nutmeg

- **Ingredients**: 1 cup warm milk (dairy or plant-based), a pinch of nutmeg.
- **Method**: Stir nutmeg into the warm milk and drink before bed.
- **Benefits**: Promotes relaxation and eases the body into sleep.

4. Passionflower Tea for Deep Sleep

- **Ingredients**: 1 tsp dried passionflower, 1 cup boiling water.
- **Method**: Steep the passionflower in boiling water for 10 minutes. Strain and drink.
- **Benefits**: Reduces anxiety and promotes restful sleep.

5. Valerian Root Tea

- **Ingredients**: 1/2 tsp valerian root, 1 cup boiling water.
- **Method**: Steep valerian root in boiling water for 10 minutes. Strain and sip slowly before bed.
- **Benefits**: Eases insomnia and calms the mind.

6. Banana and Almond Smoothie

- **Ingredients**: 1 banana, 1/2 cup almond milk, 1 tsp honey.
- **Method**: Blend all ingredients into a smooth drink and consume an hour before bedtime.
- **Benefits**: Provides magnesium and tryptophan, which promote better sleep.

7. Lavender Foot Soak

- **Ingredients**: 1/4 cup Epsom salt, 3 drops lavender essential oil, warm water.
- **Method**: Dissolve Epsom salt and lavender oil in warm water. Soak your feet for 15–20 minutes.
- **Benefits**: Relaxes the body and prepares it for sleep.

8. Holy Basil Tonic for Rest

- **Ingredients**: 1 tsp dried holy basil leaves, 1 cup boiling water.
- **Method**: Steep the leaves in boiling water for 10 minutes. Strain and drink.
- **Benefits**: Reduces stress hormones and promotes mental calmness.

9. Peppermint Steam for Relaxation

- **Ingredients**: 2 drops peppermint essential oil, bowl of hot water.
- **Method**: Add peppermint oil to the water, cover your head with a towel, and inhale the steam deeply.
- **Benefits**: Clears the mind and relaxes the body.

10. Rose Petal Bath Soak

- **Ingredients**: 1/2 cup fresh rose petals, warm bathwater.
- **Method**: Add rose petals to the bathwater and soak for 20 minutes before bed.
- **Benefits**: Calms the senses and reduces stress.

11. Lemon Balm Tea

- **Ingredients**: 1 tsp dried lemon balm, 1 cup boiling water.
- **Method**: Steep lemon balm in boiling water for 10 minutes. Strain and drink.
- **Benefits**: Relieves anxiety and promotes a sense of calm.

12. Frankincense Diffuser Blend

- **Ingredients**: 3 drops frankincense essential oil, a diffuser, water.
- **Method**: Add the oil to a diffuser filled with water and let it run as you prepare for bed.
- **Benefits**: Promotes grounding and relaxation.

13. Green Tea Ice Cubes for Tension Relief

- **Ingredients**: 1 cup green tea, ice cube tray.
- **Method**: Freeze brewed green tea in an ice tray and rub one cube on your face or neck.
- **Benefits**: Refreshes and soothes tension.

14. Lavender Herbal Sachet

- **Ingredients**: 1/4 cup dried lavender, a small muslin bag.
- **Method**: Place lavender in the muslin bag and keep it under your pillow.
- **Benefits**: Releases a calming scent to improve sleep quality.

15. Cinnamon and Honey Sleep Tonic

- **Ingredients**: 1/4 tsp cinnamon powder, 1 tsp honey, 1 cup warm water.
- **Method**: Mix all ingredients and drink before bed.
- **Benefits**: Relaxes the body and reduces nighttime cravings.

16. Chamomile and Fennel Digestive Tea

- **Ingredients**: 1 tsp dried chamomile, 1/2 tsp fennel seeds, 1 cup boiling water.
- **Method**: Steep ingredients in boiling water for 10 minutes. Strain and sip slowly.
- **Benefits**: Eases digestive stress and promotes calmness.

17. Aloe Vera and Mint Cooling Gel

- **Ingredients**: 2 tbsp aloe vera gel, 1 tsp crushed mint leaves.
- **Method**: Mix and apply to the skin before bedtime.
- **Benefits**: Cools and calms the skin, aiding relaxation.

18. Ylang-Ylang and Sandalwood Oil Blend

- **Ingredients**: 3 drops ylang-ylang oil, 3 drops sandalwood oil, 2 tbsp carrier oil.
- **Method**: Mix and massage onto your chest or temples before bed.
- **Benefits**: Promotes emotional balance and relaxation.

19. Warm Oatmeal Drink

- **Ingredients**: 2 tbsp oats, 1 cup warm milk, 1 tsp honey.
- **Method**: Cook oats in milk, stir in honey, and drink warm.
- **Benefits**: Encourages relaxation with its natural calming properties.

20. Magnesium Oil Spray

- **Ingredients**: 1/4 cup magnesium oil, spray bottle.
- **Method**: Spray onto your legs and feet before bed. Massage gently.
- **Benefits**: Relieves tension and promotes better sleep.

21. Blackout Curtains for Better Sleep Environment

- **Ingredients**: Blackout curtains.
- **Method**: Install in your bedroom to block out light and create a sleep-friendly environment.
- **Benefits**: Encourages deeper and uninterrupted sleep.

22. Warm Peppermint Foot Rub

- **Ingredients**: 2 drops peppermint oil, 1 tsp coconut oil.
- **Method**: Mix and massage into your feet before bedtime.
- **Benefits**: Soothes the body and calms the mind.

23. Weighted Blanket

- **Ingredients**: A weighted blanket.
- **Method**: Use a weighted blanket during sleep to feel gently compressed.
- **Benefits**: Reduces anxiety and promotes deep relaxation.

24. Cardamom Milk

- **Ingredients**: 1/4 tsp cardamom powder, 1 cup warm milk.
- **Method**: Mix cardamom into warm milk and drink before bed.
- **Benefits**: Soothes the digestive system and calms the mind.

25. Cedarwood Essential Oil for Restful Sleep

- **Ingredients**: 3 drops cedarwood essential oil, diffuser.
- **Method**: Add cedarwood oil to a diffuser and let it run as you prepare for sleep.
- **Benefits**: Relieves tension and enhances deep sleep.

26. Flaxseed and Honey Drink

- **Ingredients**: 1 tbsp flaxseed meal, 1 tsp honey, 1 cup warm water.
- **Method**: Mix flaxseed and honey into warm water and sip slowly.
- **Benefits**: Relaxes muscles and promotes restfulness.

27. Peppermint and Eucalyptus Steam

- **Ingredients**: 1 drop eucalyptus oil, 1 drop peppermint oil, bowl of hot water.
- **Method**: Add oils to hot water, inhale deeply for 5 minutes.
- **Benefits**: Clears airways and relaxes the mind.

28. Rose and Honey Mask

- **Ingredients**: 1 tbsp crushed rose petals, 1 tsp honey.

- **Method**: Mix and apply to the face before bed. Rinse after 15 minutes.
- **Benefits**: Hydrates and soothes the skin, promoting relaxation.

29. Clary Sage Diffuser Blend

- **Ingredients**: 3 drops clary sage essential oil, water, diffuser.
- **Method**: Add clary sage to your diffuser and run it in your bedroom.
- **Benefits**: Relaxes the mind and encourages sleep.

30. Banana Peel Tea

- **Ingredients**: 1 banana peel, 1 cup boiling water.
- **Method**: Boil the banana peel in water for 10 minutes, strain, and sip.
- **Benefits**: High in magnesium, it calms the body and promotes deep sleep.

Focus and Mood Boosting

1. Peppermint Tea for Mental Clarity

- **Ingredients**: 1 tsp dried peppermint leaves, 1 cup boiling water.
- **Method**: Steep peppermint leaves in boiling water for 10 minutes. Strain and sip.
- **Benefits**: Stimulates the mind, improves focus, and reduces mental fatigue.

2. Lemon Water for Fresh Energy

- **Ingredients**: Juice of 1/2 lemon, 1 cup cold water.
- **Method**: Mix lemon juice in cold water and drink in the morning or mid-afternoon.
- **Benefits**: Refreshes and energizes, while hydrating the body and improving alertness.

3. Holy Basil Tea for Emotional Balance

- **Ingredients**: 1 tsp dried holy basil leaves, 1 cup boiling water.
- **Method**: Steep the basil leaves in boiling water for 10 minutes. Strain and drink.
- **Benefits**: Balances stress hormones and enhances mental clarity.

4. Rosemary Diffuser Blend for Concentration

- **Ingredients**: 3 drops rosemary essential oil, a diffuser, water.

- **Method**: Add rosemary oil to a diffuser filled with water and let it run during work or study.
- **Benefits**: Improves memory and sharpens focus.

5. Dark Chocolate for Mental Boost

- **Ingredients**: 1 small piece of dark chocolate (70% or higher).
- **Method**: Eat slowly and savor the flavor for a mindful snack.
- **Benefits**: Contains flavonoids that improve cognitive performance and mood.

6. Peppermint and Lemon Essential Oil Mist

- **Ingredients**: 1/2 cup water, 2 drops peppermint oil, 2 drops lemon oil, spray bottle.
- **Method**: Mix all ingredients in a spray bottle and mist your workspace.
- **Benefits**: Refreshes the mind, clears mental fog, and boosts energy.

7. Matcha Tea for Sustained Energy

- **Ingredients**: 1 tsp matcha powder, 1 cup hot water, honey (optional).
- **Method**: Whisk matcha powder into hot water until frothy. Sweeten with honey if desired.
- **Benefits**: Provides a steady, caffeine-driven focus without jitters.

8. Ginseng Tonic for Alertness

- **Ingredients**: 1/2 tsp ginseng powder, 1 cup warm water, 1 tsp honey.
- **Method**: Mix the ginseng powder and honey into warm water and sip slowly.
- **Benefits**: Boosts energy levels and enhances mental clarity.

9. Orange Peel and Cinnamon Tea

- **Ingredients**: 1 tbsp dried orange peel, 1/2 cinnamon stick, 1 cup boiling water.
- **Method**: Simmer ingredients in water for 5 minutes, strain, and drink.
- **Benefits**: Uplifts mood and enhances focus with a warming, citrusy aroma.

10. Beetroot Smoothie for Brainpower

- **Ingredients**: 1/2 cup beetroot, 1/2 cup orange juice, 1/2 cup water.
- **Method**: Blend all ingredients into a smoothie and drink fresh.
- **Benefits**: Increases blood flow to the brain, enhancing focus and stamina.

11. Pineapple and Ginger Juice for Vitality

- **Ingredients**: 1 cup pineapple chunks, 1-inch ginger root, 1/2 cup water.
- **Method**: Blend the ingredients into a juice and strain if needed.
- **Benefits**: Combines antioxidants and enzymes to energize and uplift mood.

12. Green Tea with Mint for Refreshment

- **Ingredients**: 1 cup brewed green tea, 1 tsp crushed mint leaves.
- **Method**: Brew green tea, steep mint leaves in it for 5 minutes, strain, and sip.
- **Benefits**: Improves alertness and refreshes the mind.

13. Clary Sage Essential Oil for Emotional Lift

- **Ingredients**: 2 drops clary sage essential oil, 1 tsp carrier oil (e.g., coconut oil).
- **Method**: Mix oils and apply to your wrists or temples during moments of stress.
- **Benefits**: Relieves tension and balances mood swings.

14. Banana and Walnut Energy Snack

- **Ingredients**: 1 banana, 2 tbsp crushed walnuts.
- **Method**: Slice the banana and sprinkle with crushed walnuts. Eat as a snack.
- **Benefits**: Combines potassium and omega-3s to boost brain function.

15. Lavender and Rosemary Sachet for Focus

- **Ingredients**: 1 tbsp dried lavender, 1 tbsp dried rosemary, a small muslin bag.
- **Method**: Combine lavender and rosemary in the muslin bag and keep it on your desk.
- **Benefits**: Provides calming yet invigorating scents to boost focus.

16. Lemon and Ginger Detox Water

- **Ingredients**: 3 lemon slices, 1-inch ginger root (sliced), 1 liter water.
- **Method**: Add lemon and ginger slices to water and let infuse for 1 hour. Sip throughout the day.
- **Benefits**: Cleanses toxins and refreshes the mind and body.

17. Sage and Thyme Steam Inhalation

- **Ingredients**: 1 tsp dried sage, 1 tsp dried thyme, bowl of hot water.
- **Method**: Add herbs to the bowl of hot water, cover your head with a towel, and inhale deeply.

- **Benefits**: Improves focus and clears mental fog.

18. Orange and Rosehip Tea

- **Ingredients**: 1 tsp dried rosehips, 1 tsp dried orange peel, 1 cup boiling water.
- **Method**: Steep both in boiling water for 10 minutes, strain, and drink.
- **Benefits**: Boosts mood and refreshes the senses.

19. Basil and Mint Cooler

- **Ingredients**: 5 fresh basil leaves, 5 fresh mint leaves, 1 cup cold water.
- **Method**: Muddle the herbs, add to cold water, and let infuse for 30 minutes.
- **Benefits**: Clears mental fatigue and energizes the body.

20. Peppermint Chocolate Energy Drink

- **Ingredients**: 1 cup warm milk, 1 tbsp dark cocoa powder, 1 drop peppermint oil.
- **Method**: Mix all ingredients and sip warm.
- **Benefits**: Combines chocolate's mood-boosting properties with peppermint's mental clarity benefits.

21. Almond and Honey Snack

- **Ingredients**: 10 almonds, 1 tsp honey.
- **Method**: Drizzle honey over almonds and eat as a quick snack.
- **Benefits**: Provides sustained energy and brain-nourishing nutrients.

22. Ginger and Turmeric Tea

- **Ingredients**: 1-inch ginger root, 1/2 tsp turmeric, 1 cup boiling water.
- **Method**: Simmer ginger and turmeric in water for 5 minutes, strain, and drink.
- **Benefits**: Combats fatigue and inflammation while uplifting mood.

23. Blueberry and Spinach Smoothie

- **Ingredients**: 1/2 cup blueberries, 1/2 cup spinach, 1 cup water.
- **Method**: Blend all ingredients into a smoothie and drink fresh.
- **Benefits**: Improves cognitive function and provides antioxidants.

24. Cinnamon and Apple Tea

- **Ingredients**: 1/2 apple (sliced), 1/2 cinnamon stick, 1 cup boiling water.
- **Method**: Simmer apple and cinnamon in boiling water for 10 minutes. Strain and drink.
- **Benefits**: Boosts mood and sharpens focus with comforting aromas.

25. Lavender and Lemon Oil Diffuser Blend

- **Ingredients**: 3 drops lavender oil, 3 drops lemon oil, a diffuser.
- **Method**: Add oils to your diffuser and let the blend permeate your space.
- **Benefits**: Reduces stress while uplifting energy and focus.

26. Avocado Toast with Chili Flakes

- **Ingredients**: 1 slice whole-grain bread, 1/2 avocado, pinch of chili flakes.
- **Method**: Spread mashed avocado on toast, sprinkle chili flakes, and eat fresh.
- **Benefits**: Provides healthy fats for brain health and a spicy kick for alertness.

27. Lemon Balm and Honey Tea

- **Ingredients**: 1 tsp dried lemon balm, 1 tsp honey, 1 cup boiling water.
- **Method**: Steep lemon balm in boiling water for 10 minutes. Stir in honey and drink.
- **Benefits**: Calms the nerves while improving mood and mental clarity.

28. Peppermint Scalp Massage Oil

- **Ingredients**: 2 drops peppermint oil, 1 tsp coconut oil.
- **Method**: Mix and massage onto your scalp for 5–10 minutes.
- **Benefits**: Improves blood flow and energizes the mind.

29. Pomegranate Juice for Brainpower

- **Ingredients**: 1 cup fresh pomegranate juice.
- **Method**: Drink chilled or at room temperature as a midday refreshment.
- **Benefits**: Improves blood flow to the brain and enhances mood.

30. Cardamom and Ginger Tea

- **Ingredients**: 2 cardamom pods, 1-inch ginger root, 1 cup boiling water.
- **Method**: Simmer cardamom and ginger in water for 5 minutes, strain, and drink.

- **Benefits**: Relieves fatigue and boosts mental energy.

3.4 Immune Support and Prevention

Immune Boosters

1. Astragalus Tea for Long-Term Immune Strength

- **Ingredients**: 1 tsp dried astragalus root, 2 cups water.
- **Method**: Simmer astragalus root in water for 20 minutes. Strain and drink daily.
- **Benefits**: Supports long-term immune health and helps prevent infections.

2. Black Seed Oil Tonic to Fight Inflammation

- **Ingredients**: 1 tsp black seed oil, 1/2 cup warm water, 1 tsp honey.
- **Method**: Mix black seed oil and honey into warm water and drink on an empty stomach.
- **Benefits**: Reduces chronic inflammation and enhances immune resilience.

3. Reishi Mushroom Tea to Enhance Immune Response

- **Ingredients**: 1 tsp dried reishi mushroom powder, 2 cups water.
- **Method**: Simmer mushroom powder in water for 30 minutes, strain, and drink.
- **Benefits**: Modulates the immune system and reduces oxidative stress.

4. Fermented Garlic for Natural Antibiotic Support

- **Ingredients**: 10 garlic cloves, 1/4 cup raw honey.
- **Method**: Slightly crush garlic cloves, submerge them in honey, and ferment for 5 days. Consume 1 clove daily.
- **Benefits**: Acts as a natural antibiotic and strengthens immunity.

5. Spirulina Lemon Drink for Antioxidant Boost

- **Ingredients**: 1 tsp spirulina powder, juice of 1/2 lemon, 1 cup water.
- **Method**: Mix spirulina and lemon into water, stir well, and drink.
- **Benefits**: Provides antioxidants that boost immune cell production.

6. Ginger-Turmeric Shot to Combat Infections

- **Ingredients**: 1-inch ginger, 1/2 tsp turmeric, 1/4 tsp black pepper, 1/2 cup water.
- **Method**: Blend into a shot and drink in the morning.
- **Benefits**: Combats infections and reduces inflammation.

7. Herbal Vinegar Infusion for Antimicrobial Defense

- **Ingredients**: 1 cup raw apple cider vinegar, 1 tbsp dried rosemary, 1 tbsp thyme.
- **Method**: Steep herbs in vinegar for 2 weeks, strain, and take 1 tbsp diluted in water daily.
- **Benefits**: Provides antimicrobial properties that protect against infections.

8. Probiotic Pickled Vegetables to Strengthen Gut Immunity

- **Ingredients**: 2 cups chopped vegetables (carrots, cucumbers, radishes), 1 tbsp sea salt, 2 cups water.
- **Method**: Dissolve salt in water, pour over vegetables in a jar, and ferment for 1–2 weeks.
- **Benefits**: Boosts gut health, which is critical for a strong immune system.

9. Echinacea Tea for Preventing Colds

- **Ingredients**: 1 tsp dried echinacea, 1 cup boiling water.
- **Method**: Steep echinacea in boiling water for 10 minutes, strain, and drink.
- **Benefits**: Helps prevent and reduce the duration of colds.

10. Tulsi Tea for Respiratory Immunity

- **Ingredients**: 1 tsp dried tulsi leaves, 1 cup boiling water.
- **Method**: Steep tulsi leaves in boiling water for 10 minutes. Strain and drink.
- **Benefits**: Improves respiratory immunity and fights infections.

11. Amla Juice for Vitamin C Boost

- **Ingredients**: 1 tbsp amla (Indian gooseberry) powder, 1 cup water.
- **Method**: Mix amla powder into water, stir, and drink daily.
- **Benefits**: Provides high levels of vitamin C to support the immune system.

12. Licorice Root Tea for Respiratory Protection

- **Ingredients**: 1 tbsp licorice root, 2 cups water, 1 tsp honey.
- **Method**: Simmer licorice root in water for 15 minutes, strain, and sweeten with honey.

- **Benefits**: Soothes the throat and enhances respiratory immunity.

13. Pine Needle Tea for Viral Defense

- **Ingredients**: 1 tsp dried pine needles, 1 cup boiling water.
- **Method**: Steep pine needles in boiling water for 10 minutes, strain, and sip.
- **Benefits**: Supports the immune system with antiviral compounds.

14. Wheatgrass Shot for Cellular Immunity

- **Ingredients**: 1/2 cup fresh wheatgrass, 1/4 cup water.
- **Method**: Blend wheatgrass with water, strain, and drink as a shot.
- **Benefits**: Detoxifies the body and boosts cellular immunity.

15. Herbal Immune Syrup for Daily Support

- **Ingredients**: 1/2 cup elderberries, 1/4 cup dried rosehips, 2 cups water, 1/2 cup honey.
- **Method**: Simmer elderberries and rosehips in water for 30 minutes. Strain, cool, and add honey. Take 1 tbsp daily.
- **Benefits**: Combines antiviral and immune-strengthening properties.

16. Moringa Leaf Tea for Overall Immune Boost

- **Ingredients**: 1 tsp dried moringa leaves, 1 cup boiling water.
- **Method**: Steep leaves in boiling water for 10 minutes, strain, and drink.
- **Benefits**: Packed with nutrients that support immune function.

17. Black Pepper and Honey Mix for Cold Prevention

- **Ingredients**: 1/4 tsp black pepper powder, 1 tsp honey.
- **Method**: Mix and consume daily.
- **Benefits**: Antibacterial and helps prevent respiratory infections.

18. Beetroot and Carrot Smoothie for Antioxidants

- **Ingredients**: 1/2 cup beetroot, 1/2 cup carrots, 1/4 cup orange juice.
- **Method**: Blend into a smoothie and drink fresh.
- **Benefits**: Provides antioxidants that strengthen immunity.

19. Golden Milk for Anti-Inflammatory Support

- **Ingredients**: 1 cup milk (dairy or plant-based), 1/2 tsp turmeric, 1/4 tsp black pepper.
- **Method**: Heat milk, mix in turmeric and black pepper, and drink warm.
- **Benefits**: Combines anti-inflammatory properties with immune-boosting benefits.

20. Probiotic Yogurt to Support Gut Health

- **Ingredients**: 1 cup plain probiotic yogurt.
- **Method**: Eat daily as a snack or part of a meal.
- **Benefits**: Enhances gut microbiome health, which is key to immune function.

21. Ginger Garlic Paste for Infection Defense

- **Ingredients**: 1-inch ginger, 3 garlic cloves, 1 tsp olive oil.
- **Method**: Blend ginger and garlic into a paste. Use as a seasoning in soups or broths.
- **Benefits**: Combines antimicrobial and immune-boosting properties.

22. Cinnamon and Clove Tea for Antiviral Protection

- **Ingredients**: 1/2 tsp cinnamon, 2 cloves, 1 cup boiling water.
- **Method**: Simmer spices in water for 10 minutes, strain, and drink.
- **Benefits**: Provides antiviral properties that strengthen immunity.

23. Ashwagandha Root Infusion for Stress-Resilient Immunity

- **Ingredients**: 1 tsp dried ashwagandha root, 2 cups water, 1 tsp honey (optional).
- **Method**: Simmer ashwagandha root in water for 15–20 minutes. Strain, sweeten with honey if desired, and drink.
- **Benefits**: An adaptogen that reduces stress, enhances immune response, and strengthens the body's resistance to illnesses.

24. Aloe Vera Juice for Digestive and Immune Support

- **Ingredients**: 2 tbsp fresh aloe vera gel, 1 cup water, 1 tsp lemon juice.
- **Method**: Blend aloe vera gel with water and lemon juice. Drink fresh on an empty stomach.
- **Benefits**: Soothes the gut, reduces inflammation, and boosts the immune system by promoting better digestion and detoxification.

25. Nigella Seeds Paste for Antiviral Support

- **Ingredients**: 1 tsp nigella (black cumin) seeds, 1 tsp honey.
- **Method**: Grind the nigella seeds into a powder and mix with honey to make a paste. Consume 1 tsp daily.
- **Benefits**: Boosts immune response and provides antiviral and antibacterial benefits.

26. Shatavari Powder Drink for Hormonal and Immune Balance

- **Ingredients**: 1 tsp shatavari powder, 1 cup warm milk (dairy or plant-based), 1/2 tsp honey.
- **Method**: Stir shatavari powder and honey into warm milk and drink before bed.
- **Benefits**: Enhances immunity, balances hormones, and supports overall vitality, especially for women.

27. Mushroom Broth for Immune Cell Activation

- **Ingredients**: 1/2 cup shiitake or maitake mushrooms, 4 cups water, 1 tsp ginger (grated).
- **Method**: Simmer mushrooms and ginger in water for 30 minutes. Strain and drink as a warm broth.
- **Benefits**: Activates immune cells and enhances the body's defense mechanisms.

28. Dry Brushing for Lymphatic Drainage and Detox

- **Ingredients**: A natural bristle brush.
- **Method**: Gently brush the skin in circular motions, starting from your feet and moving upward toward your heart, for 5–10 minutes daily before showering.
- **Benefits**: Stimulates the lymphatic system, removes toxins, and supports immunity by improving circulation.

29. Cabbage and Apple Fermented Slaw for Probiotic Support

- **Ingredients**: 1 cup shredded cabbage, 1/2 grated apple, 1 tsp sea salt.
- **Method**: Mix all ingredients in a clean jar, press firmly to release juices, and cover. Let ferment for 5–7 days. Consume 1–2 tbsp daily.
- **Benefits**: Provides probiotics that enhance gut health and strengthen the immune system.

30. Bay Leaf Infusion for Respiratory Defense

- **Ingredients**: 2 dried bay leaves, 1 cup boiling water.
- **Method**: Steep bay leaves in boiling water for 10 minutes. Strain and sip slowly.

- **Benefits**: Clears congestion, improves respiratory health, and strengthens immunity with antimicrobial properties.

Antiviral and Antimicrobial Solutions

1. Garlic Honey Syrup for Fighting Viruses

- **Ingredients**: 5 garlic cloves (crushed), 1/4 cup raw honey.
- **Method**: Combine garlic and honey in a jar. Let it infuse for 2 days, then take 1 tsp daily.
- **Benefits**: Acts as a natural antibiotic, fighting bacteria and viruses effectively.

2. Thyme Steam for Clearing Respiratory Infections

- **Ingredients**: 1 tsp dried thyme, 1 bowl of hot water.
- **Method**: Add thyme to hot water, cover your head with a towel, and inhale deeply for 10 minutes.
- **Benefits**: Clears congestion and fights respiratory infections with strong antimicrobial properties.

3. Clove Oil Mouth Rinse for Oral Bacteria

- **Ingredients**: 1 drop clove essential oil, 1/2 cup warm water.
- **Method**: Mix clove oil with warm water and use as a mouth rinse twice daily.
- **Benefits**: Kills oral bacteria, freshens breath, and prevents infections.

4. Neem Water Wash for Skin Infections

- **Ingredients**: 1/4 cup neem leaves, 1 liter water.
- **Method**: Boil neem leaves in water for 10 minutes, strain, and use the water to wash infected skin.
- **Benefits**: Antifungal and antibacterial, it helps treat skin infections naturally.

5. Ginger Tea for Viral Fevers

- **Ingredients**: 1-inch ginger (sliced), 1 cup boiling water, 1 tsp honey.
- **Method**: Steep ginger in boiling water for 10 minutes. Strain, add honey, and drink warm.
- **Benefits**: Fights viruses, reduces fever, and soothes the throat.

6. Eucalyptus Oil Steam for Sinus Infections

- **Ingredients**: 3 drops eucalyptus oil, bowl of hot water.

- **Method**: Add eucalyptus oil to hot water, cover your head with a towel, and inhale deeply for 5–10 minutes.
- **Benefits**: Opens nasal passages and kills bacteria in the sinuses.

7. Apple Cider Vinegar Rinse for Fungal Infections

- **Ingredients**: 1/2 cup apple cider vinegar, 1 cup warm water.
- **Method**: Mix and use as a rinse on affected skin or scalp.
- **Benefits**: Antifungal properties help fight infections like athlete's foot or dandruff.

8. Black Cumin Seeds for Immunity

- **Ingredients**: 1 tsp black cumin seeds, 1 tsp honey.
- **Method**: Mix seeds with honey and consume daily.
- **Benefits**: Antiviral and antibacterial properties support overall immunity.

9. Peppermint Tea for Digestive Viruses

- **Ingredients**: 1 tsp dried peppermint leaves, 1 cup boiling water.
- **Method**: Steep peppermint leaves in boiling water for 10 minutes. Strain and sip warm.
- **Benefits**: Fights digestive infections and soothes upset stomachs.

10. Turmeric Paste for Skin Wounds

- **Ingredients**: 1 tsp turmeric powder, a few drops of water.
- **Method**: Mix into a paste and apply to cuts or wounds. Cover with a clean bandage.
- **Benefits**: Prevents infections and speeds up wound healing.

11. Basil Tea for Viral Colds

- **Ingredients**: 1 tsp dried basil leaves, 1 cup boiling water.
- **Method**: Steep basil leaves in boiling water for 10 minutes. Strain and drink warm.
- **Benefits**: Reduces cold symptoms and fights respiratory viruses.

12. Oregano Oil Capsules for Bacterial Infections

- **Ingredients**: 1 oregano oil capsule.
- **Method**: Take 1 capsule daily with water (consult a doctor for dosage).
- **Benefits**: Potent antimicrobial properties fight internal bacterial infections.

13. Onion Compress for Ear Infections

- **Ingredients**: 1 onion (sliced).
- **Method**: Heat the onion slices slightly, wrap them in a cloth, and apply to the ear for 10 minutes.
- **Benefits**: Draws out infection and reduces pain naturally.

14. Fenugreek Seed Tea for Infections

- **Ingredients**: 1 tsp fenugreek seeds, 1 cup boiling water.
- **Method**: Simmer seeds in water for 10 minutes, strain, and drink.
- **Benefits**: Antiviral and antibacterial properties fight internal infections.

15. Lemon and Honey Gargle for Sore Throats

- **Ingredients**: Juice of 1/2 lemon, 1 tsp honey, 1/2 cup warm water.
- **Method**: Mix and gargle for 2 minutes.
- **Benefits**: Soothes sore throats and kills bacteria in the mouth and throat.

16. Calendula Salve for Skin Infections

- **Ingredients**: 1/4 cup calendula oil, 1 tbsp beeswax.
- **Method**: Melt beeswax, mix with calendula oil, and cool. Apply to infected skin twice daily.
- **Benefits**: Antimicrobial and anti-inflammatory for skin healing.

17. Clove and Turmeric Toothpaste for Gum Health

- **Ingredients**: 1/2 tsp clove powder, 1/4 tsp turmeric, 1 tsp coconut oil.
- **Method**: Mix into a paste and brush your teeth with it.
- **Benefits**: Antibacterial properties fight gum infections and prevent tooth decay.

18. Witch Hazel Spray for Fungal Infections

- **Ingredients**: 1/2 cup witch hazel, 5 drops tea tree oil.
- **Method**: Mix and spray on infected skin twice daily.
- **Benefits**: Kills fungal spores and prevents further spread.

19. Lemon Balm Tea for Herpes Viruses

- **Ingredients**: 1 tsp dried lemon balm, 1 cup boiling water.

- **Method**: Steep lemon balm in boiling water for 10 minutes. Strain and drink.
- **Benefits**: Antiviral properties help suppress herpes outbreaks.

20. Tea Tree Oil Nail Solution for Fungus

- **Ingredients**: 1 drop tea tree oil, 1 tsp carrier oil (coconut or olive oil).
- **Method**: Mix and apply to infected nails twice daily.
- **Benefits**: Treats nail fungus and prevents its spread.

21. Rosemary Steam for Antiviral Protection

- **Ingredients**: 1 tsp dried rosemary, bowl of hot water.
- **Method**: Add rosemary to hot water, cover your head with a towel, and inhale deeply.
- **Benefits**: Clears respiratory passages and fights airborne viruses.

22. Garlic Oil for Ear Infections

- **Ingredients**: 1 clove garlic (crushed), 1 tbsp olive oil.
- **Method**: Warm garlic in olive oil, strain, and use 2–3 drops in the affected ear.
- **Benefits**: Antibacterial and antiviral properties fight ear infections.

23. Sage Gargle for Mouth Ulcers

- **Ingredients**: 1 tsp dried sage, 1 cup boiling water.
- **Method**: Steep sage in boiling water for 10 minutes, strain, and use as a gargle.
- **Benefits**: Heals mouth ulcers and fights bacteria in the mouth.

24. Coconut Oil Rub for Bacterial Skin Infections

- **Ingredients**: 1 tbsp coconut oil.
- **Method**: Massage coconut oil onto infected areas of the skin twice daily.
- **Benefits**: Antibacterial and moisturizing for infected or inflamed skin.

25. Propolis Tincture for Wound Healing

- **Ingredients**: 2–3 drops propolis tincture.
- **Method**: Apply directly to wounds or sores.
- **Benefits**: Antiviral and antibacterial for faster healing.

26. Black Tea Compress for Viral Pink Eye

- **Ingredients**: 1 black tea bag, 1/2 cup warm water.
- **Method**: Soak tea bag in warm water, cool slightly, and place on the infected eye for 10 minutes.
- **Benefits**: Reduces inflammation and fights viral eye infections.

27. Bay Leaf Tea for Antiviral Support

- **Ingredients**: 2 dried bay leaves, 1 cup boiling water.
- **Method**: Steep bay leaves in boiling water for 10 minutes. Strain and drink.
- **Benefits**: Contains antiviral compounds that help the body fight against colds, flu, and other infections.

28. Manuka Honey for Wound Infections

- **Ingredients**: 1 tsp Manuka honey.
- **Method**: Apply a thin layer of Manuka honey directly to a wound or infected area. Cover with a clean bandage.
- **Benefits**: Manuka honey's strong antimicrobial properties help heal wounds and prevent infection.

29. Thyme Oil Chest Rub for Respiratory Viruses

- **Ingredients**: 3 drops thyme essential oil, 1 tbsp coconut oil.
- **Method**: Mix oils and rub on the chest before sleep.
- **Benefits**: Opens airways, reduces cough, and fights respiratory infections caused by viruses and bacteria.

30. Elderberry Lozenges for Viral Relief

- **Ingredients**: 1/4 cup elderberry syrup, 1/4 cup honey, 1/4 tsp cinnamon powder, silicone mold.
- **Method**: Mix elderberry syrup, honey, and cinnamon. Pour into molds and freeze until solid. Suck on lozenges as needed.
- **Benefits**: Elderberry helps reduce the duration of colds and flu while providing antiviral support.

Everyday Prevention

1. Lemon and Honey Morning Tonic

- **Ingredients**: Juice of 1/2 lemon, 1 tsp honey, 1 cup warm water.
- **Method**: Mix and drink on an empty stomach every morning.
- **Benefits**: Boosts digestion, detoxifies, and strengthens immunity.

2. Turmeric Milk for Nightly Recovery

- **Ingredients**: 1 cup warm milk (dairy or plant-based), 1/2 tsp turmeric powder, 1/4 tsp black pepper.
- **Method**: Mix turmeric and black pepper into milk. Drink before bed.
- **Benefits**: Reduces inflammation, supports immunity, and aids restful sleep.

3. Apple Cider Vinegar Daily Detox

- **Ingredients**: 1 tbsp apple cider vinegar, 1 cup warm water, 1 tsp honey (optional).
- **Method**: Stir apple cider vinegar into warm water. Drink before meals.
- **Benefits**: Balances gut pH, supports digestion, and prevents infections.

4. Holy Basil (Tulsi) Tea

- **Ingredients**: 1 tsp dried tulsi leaves, 1 cup boiling water.
- **Method**: Steep tulsi in boiling water for 10 minutes. Strain and sip daily.
- **Benefits**: Reduces stress and boosts respiratory health.

5. Morning Stretch Routine

- **Ingredients**: None.
- **Method**: Dedicate 10 minutes each morning to stretching, focusing on major muscle groups.
- **Benefits**: Improves circulation, flexibility, and mental clarity.

6. Spirulina and Lemon Immunity Booster

- **Ingredients**: 1 tsp spirulina powder, juice of 1/2 lemon, 1 cup water.
- **Method**: Mix spirulina and lemon into water. Stir well and drink daily.
- **Benefits**: Packed with antioxidants, vitamins, and immune-boosting nutrients.

7. Epsom Salt Bath for Detox

- **Ingredients**: 1 cup Epsom salt, warm bathwater.
- **Method**: Dissolve Epsom salt in bathwater and soak for 20 minutes weekly.
- **Benefits**: Draws out toxins, relaxes muscles, and reduces stress.

8. Ginger and Cinnamon Morning Tonic

- **Ingredients**: 1-inch ginger (sliced), 1/2 cinnamon stick, 1 cup boiling water.
- **Method**: Steep ginger and cinnamon in boiling water for 10 minutes. Strain and drink.
- **Benefits**: Stimulates digestion, boosts circulation, and prevents colds.

9. Green Tea with Mint

- **Ingredients**: 1 green tea bag, 1 tsp fresh mint leaves, 1 cup boiling water.
- **Method**: Brew green tea with mint leaves. Drink warm.
- **Benefits**: Improves focus, fights free radicals, and supports digestion.

10. Dry Brushing for Lymphatic Health

- **Ingredients**: A natural bristle brush.
- **Method**: Gently brush the skin in upward motions before a shower.
- **Benefits**: Stimulates lymphatic drainage, detoxifies, and improves skin texture.

11. Cumin, Coriander, and Fennel Tea

- **Ingredients**: 1 tsp cumin seeds, 1 tsp coriander seeds, 1 tsp fennel seeds, 3 cups water.
- **Method**: Simmer seeds in water for 10 minutes. Strain and drink throughout the day.
- **Benefits**: Balances digestion and boosts overall wellness.

12. Deep Breathing Exercise

- **Ingredients**: None.
- **Method**: Practice diaphragmatic breathing for 5 minutes daily. Inhale deeply, hold for a few seconds, and exhale slowly.
- **Benefits**: Reduces stress, improves oxygenation, and strengthens lung capacity.

13. Ashwagandha Latte for Stress Relief

- **Ingredients**: 1/2 tsp ashwagandha powder, 1 cup warm milk, 1 tsp honey.
- **Method**: Mix ashwagandha into warm milk. Drink before bedtime.
- **Benefits**: Reduces cortisol, enhances immunity, and improves sleep.

14. Probiotic-Rich Yogurt Snack

- **Ingredients**: 1 cup plain probiotic yogurt, a handful of fresh berries.
- **Method**: Combine yogurt and berries for a healthy snack.
- **Benefits**: Promotes gut health, which is closely linked to immunity.

15. Black Pepper and Honey Cough Prevention

- **Ingredients**: 1/4 tsp black pepper powder, 1 tsp honey.
- **Method**: Mix and consume daily in the morning.
- **Benefits**: Antimicrobial properties protect against throat infections.

16. Lemon Balm Tea for Calm and Focus

- **Ingredients**: 1 tsp dried lemon balm, 1 cup boiling water.
- **Method**: Steep lemon balm in boiling water for 10 minutes. Strain and drink.
- **Benefits**: Reduces stress and improves focus.

17. Pomegranate Juice for Antioxidants

- **Ingredients**: 1 cup fresh pomegranate juice.
- **Method**: Drink fresh juice daily as a mid-morning refreshment.
- **Benefits**: Rich in antioxidants that protect cells and boost immunity.

18. Curry Leaf Powder for Detox

- **Ingredients**: 1 tsp curry leaf powder, 1 cup warm water.
- **Method**: Mix curry leaf powder into warm water and drink on an empty stomach.
- **Benefits**: Detoxifies the liver and supports digestion.

19. Lemon Peel Infusion for Antioxidants

- **Ingredients**: Peel of 1 lemon, 2 cups boiling water.
- **Method**: Simmer lemon peel in water for 10 minutes, strain, and drink.
- **Benefits**: Rich in flavonoids that reduce inflammation and protect against infections.

20. Bay Leaf Tea for Respiratory Health

- **Ingredients**: 2 dried bay leaves, 1 cup boiling water.
- **Method**: Steep bay leaves in boiling water for 10 minutes. Strain and sip.
- **Benefits**: Improves respiratory health and helps prevent colds.

21. Hydration Reminder Practice

- **Ingredients**: None.
- **Method**: Set alarms or use apps to ensure you drink at least 8 glasses of water daily.
- **Benefits**: Keeps the body hydrated and flushes out toxins.

22. Fenugreek Seed Water for Blood Sugar Balance

- **Ingredients**: 1 tsp fenugreek seeds, 1 cup water.
- **Method**: Soak fenugreek seeds in water overnight. Strain and drink in the morning.
- **Benefits**: Balances blood sugar and boosts immunity.

23. Herbal Bath Soak for Stress Relief

- **Ingredients**: 1/2 cup dried chamomile, 1/4 cup dried lavender, warm bathwater.
- **Method**: Add herbs to warm water and soak for 20 minutes weekly.
- **Benefits**: Reduces stress and promotes overall relaxation.

24. Neem Leaf Tea for Skin and Immunity

- **Ingredients**: 1 tsp dried neem leaves, 1 cup boiling water.
- **Method**: Steep neem leaves in boiling water for 10 minutes. Strain and drink weekly.
- **Benefits**: Cleanses the blood and boosts immunity.

25. Morning Sunlight Exposure

- **Ingredients**: None.
- **Method**: Spend 10–15 minutes in morning sunlight daily.
- **Benefits**: Improves vitamin D levels and enhances immune function.

26. Cabbage and Carrot Slaw for Antioxidants

- **Ingredients**: 1 cup shredded cabbage, 1/2 cup shredded carrot, 1 tsp olive oil.
- **Method**: Toss all ingredients and consume as a salad.
- **Benefits**: Rich in antioxidants that prevent cellular damage.

27. Licorice Root Tea for Immune Support

- **Ingredients**: 1 tsp dried licorice root, 1 cup boiling water.

- **Method**: Steep licorice root in boiling water for 10 minutes. Strain and drink.
- **Benefits**: Soothes the throat and boosts immunity.

28. Black Sesame Seed Mix for Nutritional Balance

- **Ingredients**: 1 tbsp black sesame seeds, 1 tsp honey.
- **Method**: Mix and consume daily as a snack.
- **Benefits**: Provides healthy fats and boosts immunity.

29. Deep Sleep Hygiene Practice

- **Ingredients**: None.
- **Method**: Maintain consistent sleep patterns, avoid screens before bed, and create a calming nighttime routine.
- **Benefits**: Restores energy and strengthens the immune system.

30. Herbal Oil Massage for Circulation

- **Ingredients**: 2 tbsp sesame oil, 2 drops lavender essential oil.
- **Method**: Mix oils and massage onto the body in circular motions before a warm shower.
- **Benefits**: Improves circulation and enhances lymphatic detox.

3.5 Women's Wellness

Menstrual Health

1. Warm Castor Oil Pack for Cramps

- **Ingredients**: 2 tbsp castor oil, a soft cloth, a hot water bottle.
- **Method**: Soak the cloth in warm castor oil, apply it to the lower abdomen, and place a hot water bottle on top. Leave for 20–30 minutes.
- **Benefits**: Improves blood flow, relaxes muscles, and alleviates cramps.

2. Lavender Essential Oil Massage for Relaxation

- **Ingredients**: 2 drops lavender essential oil, 1 tsp almond oil.
- **Method**: Mix oils and massage onto the lower abdomen in circular motions.
- **Benefits**: Relaxes uterine muscles and reduces cramping and stress.

3. Epsom Salt Bath for Cramps

- **Ingredients**: 1 cup Epsom salt, warm bathwater.
- **Method**: Dissolve Epsom salt in a warm bath and soak for 20 minutes.
- **Benefits**: Relieves muscle tension and eases menstrual pain.

4. Yoga for Cramp Relief (Child's Pose)

- **Ingredients**: None.
- **Method**: Sit on your knees, stretch your arms forward, and rest your forehead on the floor. Hold for 2–3 minutes.
- **Benefits**: Relaxes the lower back and abdominal muscles.

5. Clove Oil Rub for Intense Cramps

- **Ingredients**: 1 drop clove essential oil, 1 tsp coconut oil.
- **Method**: Mix oils and rub gently onto the lower abdomen.
- **Benefits**: Provides localized pain relief with anti-inflammatory properties.

6. Fenugreek Seed Compress for Cramp Relief

- **Ingredients**: 2 tbsp fenugreek seeds, a clean cloth.
- **Method**: Boil fenugreek seeds, wrap them in a cloth, and apply to the lower abdomen.
- **Benefits**: Relieves cramps by relaxing uterine muscles.

7. Magnesium Spray for Tension Relief

- **Ingredients**: 1/4 cup magnesium oil (store-bought or homemade).
- **Method**: Spray onto the lower abdomen and gently massage.
- **Benefits**: Relaxes muscles and reduces PMS-related aches.

8. Rose Oil Diffusion for Emotional Balance

- **Ingredients**: 5 drops rose essential oil, a diffuser, water.
- **Method**: Add rose oil to a diffuser with water and run for 30 minutes.
- **Benefits**: Calms mood swings and reduces menstrual stress.

9. Warm Ginger Compress for Lower Back Pain

- **Ingredients**: 1-inch ginger (sliced), 2 cups water, a cloth.
- **Method**: Simmer ginger in water for 10 minutes, soak the cloth in the liquid, and apply to the lower back.
- **Benefits**: Reduces inflammation and alleviates back pain.

10. Vitamin B6-Rich Snack for PMS

- **Ingredients**: 1 banana, 1 tbsp almond butter.
- **Method**: Slice the banana and spread almond butter on top. Eat as a snack.
- **Benefits**: Reduces mood swings, breast tenderness, and fatigue.

11. Peppermint Essential Oil Foot Massage for Headaches

- **Ingredients**: 1 drop peppermint oil, 1 tsp carrier oil (e.g., olive oil).
- **Method**: Mix oils and massage onto the soles of the feet, focusing on the arch.
- **Benefits**: Relieves headaches associated with PMS and calms the nervous system.

12. Flaxseed Wrap for Hormonal Balance

- **Ingredients**: 2 tbsp ground flaxseeds, a clean cloth.

- **Method**: Warm the flaxseeds slightly, wrap in a cloth, and place on the lower abdomen.
- **Benefits**: Provides gentle warmth and hormone-balancing benefits.

13. Cooling Aloe Gel Rub for Breast Tenderness

- **Ingredients**: 2 tbsp aloe vera gel.
- **Method**: Apply aloe vera gel directly to the breasts and massage gently.
- **Benefits**: Reduces tenderness and soothes inflamed tissues.

14. Cumin and Salt Warm Drink for Regulating Flow

- **Ingredients**: 1 tsp cumin seeds, 1/4 tsp rock salt, 1 cup warm water.
- **Method**: Mix all ingredients and sip slowly.
- **Benefits**: Stimulates menstrual flow and eases delayed cycles.

15. Fennel Seed Porridge for Bloating

- **Ingredients**: 1 tsp fennel seeds, 1/2 cup oats, 1 cup water, 1 tsp honey.
- **Method**: Cook fennel seeds and oats in water. Sweeten with honey and eat warm.
- **Benefits**: Reduces bloating and digestive discomfort during periods.

16. Marjoram Oil Massage for Irregular Cycles

- **Ingredients**: 2 drops marjoram essential oil, 1 tsp olive oil.
- **Method**: Mix oils and massage onto the abdomen in circular motions.
- **Benefits**: Regulates menstrual cycles and reduces cramping.

17. Acupressure for Cramp Relief

- **Ingredients**: None.
- **Method**: Apply firm pressure with your thumb 3 finger-widths below your navel for 2 minutes.
- **Benefits**: Stimulates blood flow and eases cramps.

18. Papaya Smoothie for Regulating Cycles

- **Ingredients**: 1/2 cup ripe papaya, 1/2 cup almond milk, 1 tsp honey.
- **Method**: Blend all ingredients into a smoothie. Drink daily leading up to your period.
- **Benefits**: Promotes smooth menstrual flow and balances hormones.

19. Mustard Foot Soak for Full-Body Relaxation

- **Ingredients**: 2 tbsp mustard powder, warm water.
- **Method**: Add mustard powder to warm water and soak your feet for 15 minutes.
- **Benefits**: Relieves tension and improves circulation.

20. Parsley Leaf Compress for Lower Back Pain

- **Ingredients**: 1/4 cup fresh parsley leaves, a cloth.
- **Method**: Crush parsley leaves, wrap in a cloth, and place on the lower back.
- **Benefits**: Reduces inflammation and soothes back pain.

21. Sesame Oil Massage for Hormonal Balance

- **Ingredients**: 2 tbsp sesame oil.
- **Method**: Warm sesame oil and massage it onto your lower abdomen in circular motions.
- **Benefits**: Promotes hormone balance and improves circulation.

22. Licorice Root Lozenges for PMS Cravings

- **Ingredients**: 1/2 tsp licorice root powder, 1 tbsp honey.
- **Method**: Mix into a paste and roll into small lozenges. Suck on 1–2 lozenges during PMS.
- **Benefits**: Reduces sugar cravings and balances cortisol.

23. Beetroot and Carrot Compress for Pain Relief

- **Ingredients**: 1/2 cup grated beetroot, 1/2 cup grated carrot, a clean cloth.
- **Method**: Wrap the grated beetroot and carrot in the cloth and place it over the lower abdomen for 20 minutes.
- **Benefits**: Reduces cramping by improving circulation and soothing inflammation.

24. Clary Sage Oil Diffusion for Mood Swings

- **Ingredients**: 4 drops clary sage essential oil, water, a diffuser.
- **Method**: Add clary sage oil to the diffuser with water and let it run for 30 minutes in your room.
- **Benefits**: Stabilizes mood, reduces PMS-related irritability, and calms the mind.

25. Cucumber and Mint Water for Hydration and Bloating

- **Ingredients**: 1/2 cucumber (sliced), 5 mint leaves, 1 liter of water.

- **Method**: Add cucumber and mint to water and let it infuse for 1 hour. Drink throughout the day.
- **Benefits**: Reduces bloating, promotes hydration, and soothes digestive discomfort.

26. Yogurt and Turmeric Mask for Acne During Periods

- **Ingredients**: 2 tbsp plain yogurt, 1/4 tsp turmeric powder.
- **Method**: Mix yogurt and turmeric into a paste. Apply to the face, leave for 15 minutes, and rinse.
- **Benefits**: Reduces period-related acne by soothing inflammation and preventing bacterial growth.

27. Black Sesame and Jaggery Snack for Hormonal Balance

- **Ingredients**: 1 tbsp black sesame seeds, 1 tsp jaggery.
- **Method**: Mix sesame seeds and jaggery into a snack ball and consume once daily.
- **Benefits**: Regulates hormonal imbalances and supports smooth menstrual flow.

28. Aloe Vera and Coconut Oil Rub for Cramps

- **Ingredients**: 1 tbsp aloe vera gel, 1 tsp coconut oil.
- **Method**: Mix aloe vera and coconut oil. Massage onto the lower abdomen for 10 minutes.
- **Benefits**: Soothes abdominal pain and reduces inflammation.

29. Coriander Seed Water for Painful Periods

- **Ingredients**: 1 tsp coriander seeds, 1 cup boiling water.
- **Method**: Boil coriander seeds in water for 10 minutes, strain, and drink warm.
- **Benefits**: Reduces menstrual pain and promotes healthy uterine function.

30. Warm Lemon Compress for Tender Breasts

- **Ingredients**: 1/2 lemon (sliced), a clean cloth, warm water.
- **Method**: Dip the cloth in warm water, add lemon slices, and place it over the breasts for 15 minutes.
- **Benefits**: Reduces breast tenderness and improves blood flow.

Pregnancy and Postpartum Care

1. Ginger Tea for Morning Sickness

- **Ingredients**: 1-inch ginger (sliced), 1 cup boiling water.
- **Method**: Steep ginger in boiling water for 10 minutes. Strain and sip slowly.
- **Benefits**: Alleviates nausea and soothes the digestive system.

2. Lemon Water for Hydration and Fatigue

- **Ingredients**: Juice of 1/2 lemon, 1 cup warm water.
- **Method**: Mix lemon juice with warm water and drink in the morning.
- **Benefits**: Reduces morning sickness, hydrates, and boosts energy.

3. Fennel Tea for Digestion

- **Ingredients**: 1 tsp fennel seeds, 1 cup boiling water.
- **Method**: Steep fennel seeds in boiling water for 10 minutes. Strain and sip after meals.
- **Benefits**: Relieves bloating, indigestion, and gas during pregnancy.

4. Coconut Oil Massage for Stretch Marks

- **Ingredients**: 2 tbsp coconut oil.
- **Method**: Warm the oil slightly and massage onto the belly and thighs twice daily.
- **Benefits**: Moisturizes skin and improves elasticity to reduce stretch marks.

5. Peppermint Essential Oil Inhalation for Nausea

- **Ingredients**: 1 drop peppermint essential oil, a handkerchief.
- **Method**: Add the oil to a handkerchief and inhale deeply when nauseous.
- **Benefits**: Calms queasiness and boosts energy.

6. Red Raspberry Leaf Tea for Uterine Health

- **Ingredients**: 1 tsp dried red raspberry leaves, 1 cup boiling water.
- **Method**: Steep leaves in boiling water for 10 minutes. Strain and drink.
- **Benefits**: Strengthens the uterus and prepares for labor (safe in the second and third trimesters).

7. Chamomile Tea for Sleep and Anxiety

- **Ingredients**: 1 tsp dried chamomile flowers, 1 cup boiling water.
- **Method**: Steep chamomile in boiling water for 10 minutes. Strain and drink before bed.
- **Benefits**: Promotes restful sleep and reduces pregnancy-related anxiety.

8. Epsom Salt Foot Soak for Swelling

- **Ingredients**: 1/2 cup Epsom salt, warm water.
- **Method**: Dissolve Epsom salt in warm water and soak your feet for 15 minutes.
- **Benefits**: Relieves swollen feet and reduces discomfort.

9. Beetroot Juice for Energy

- **Ingredients**: 1/2 cup beetroot, 1/2 cup water.
- **Method**: Blend beetroot with water, strain, and drink fresh.
- **Benefits**: Provides iron and improves energy levels during pregnancy.

10. Almond and Date Smoothie for Energy

- **Ingredients**: 1/4 cup soaked almonds, 2 dates, 1 cup milk (dairy or plant-based).
- **Method**: Blend all ingredients into a smoothie and drink.
- **Benefits**: A rich source of energy, iron, and calcium for expectant mothers.

11. Mint and Cucumber Infused Water for Nausea

- **Ingredients**: 5 fresh mint leaves, 3 slices of cucumber, 1 liter water.
- **Method**: Add mint and cucumber to water and let it infuse for 1 hour. Sip throughout the day.
- **Benefits**: Refreshes and soothes morning sickness.

12. Lemon Balm Tea for Emotional Balance

- **Ingredients**: 1 tsp dried lemon balm, 1 cup boiling water.
- **Method**: Steep lemon balm in boiling water for 10 minutes. Strain and sip.
- **Benefits**: Reduces anxiety and stabilizes mood swings during pregnancy.

13. Dandelion Leaf Tea for Fluid Retention

- **Ingredients**: 1 tsp dried dandelion leaves, 1 cup boiling water.
- **Method**: Steep dandelion leaves in boiling water for 10 minutes. Strain and drink.
- **Benefits**: Reduces water retention and supports kidney function.

14. Flaxseed Oil for Constipation Relief

- **Ingredients**: 1 tsp flaxseed oil.
- **Method**: Take flaxseed oil once daily, mixed into oatmeal or a smoothie.
- **Benefits**: Provides fiber and promotes smooth bowel movements.

15. Prenatal Yoga for Lower Back Pain

- **Ingredients**: None.
- **Method**: Perform gentle stretches like the cat-cow pose daily.
- **Benefits**: Alleviates back pain, improves posture, and supports overall well-being.

16. Fenugreek Seed Water for Lactation Support

- **Ingredients**: 1 tsp fenugreek seeds, 1 cup water.
- **Method**: Soak fenugreek seeds in water overnight. Strain and drink in the morning.
- **Benefits**: Increases milk production and supports breastfeeding mothers.

17. Warm Compress for Breast Engorgement

- **Ingredients**: A clean cloth, warm water.
- **Method**: Soak the cloth in warm water and apply it to the breasts for 10 minutes.
- **Benefits**: Relieves engorgement and improves milk flow.

18. Turmeric Milk for Postpartum Recovery

- **Ingredients**: 1 cup warm milk, 1/2 tsp turmeric.
- **Method**: Mix turmeric into warm milk and drink before bed.
- **Benefits**: Reduces inflammation and supports faster recovery after delivery.

19. Ashwagandha Tonic for Energy

- **Ingredients**: 1/2 tsp ashwagandha powder, 1 cup warm milk, 1 tsp honey.
- **Method**: Mix ashwagandha into milk, sweeten with honey, and drink.
- **Benefits**: Restores strength, reduces stress, and improves energy.

20. Cumin Seed Water for Postpartum Cleansing

- **Ingredients**: 1 tsp cumin seeds, 1 cup water.

- **Method**: Boil cumin seeds in water for 10 minutes. Strain and sip warm.
- **Benefits**: Supports uterine health and reduces bloating after delivery.

21. Oatmeal with Brewer's Yeast for Lactation

- **Ingredients**: 1/2 cup oats, 1 tsp brewer's yeast, 1 tsp honey, 1 cup water or milk.
- **Method**: Cook oats, stir in brewer's yeast and honey, and eat warm.
- **Benefits**: Boosts milk supply and provides essential nutrients.

22. Aloe Vera Gel for Perineal Healing

- **Ingredients**: 2 tbsp fresh aloe vera gel.
- **Method**: Apply aloe vera gel gently to the perineal area after cleaning.
- **Benefits**: Soothes inflammation and speeds up healing.

23. Warm Sitz Bath for Postpartum Pain

- **Ingredients**: 1/2 cup Epsom salt, warm water.
- **Method**: Add Epsom salt to warm water in a shallow tub. Soak for 10–15 minutes.
- **Benefits**: Relieves perineal pain and reduces swelling.

24. Black Sesame and Jaggery Balls for Recovery

- **Ingredients**: 2 tbsp black sesame seeds, 1 tbsp jaggery.
- **Method**: Grind sesame seeds and jaggery together, form small balls, and eat 1 daily.
- **Benefits**: Boosts iron levels and aids postpartum recovery.

25. Lavender Oil Diffusion for Postpartum Blues

- **Ingredients**: 4 drops lavender essential oil, a diffuser, water.
- **Method**: Add lavender oil to the diffuser with water and let it run for 30 minutes.
- **Benefits**: Reduces anxiety, promotes calmness, and supports emotional balance.

26. Garlic Soup for Immunity

- **Ingredients**: 2 garlic cloves (minced), 1 cup vegetable broth.
- **Method**: Simmer garlic in broth for 10 minutes and drink warm.
- **Benefits**: Boosts immunity and aids in recovery.

27. Warm Sesame Oil Massage for Strength

- **Ingredients**: 2 tbsp sesame oil.
- **Method**: Warm the oil and gently massage your body before a shower.
- **Benefits**: Improves circulation, reduces stress, and enhances postpartum strength.

28. Holy Basil Tea for Emotional Recovery

- **Ingredients**: 1 tsp dried holy basil leaves, 1 cup boiling water.
- **Method**: Steep basil leaves in boiling water for 10 minutes. Strain and drink.
- **Benefits**: Calms the mind and supports emotional balance.

29. Cardamom Milk for Sleep

- **Ingredients**: 1 cup warm milk, 1/4 tsp cardamom powder.
- **Method**: Stir cardamom into milk and drink before bed.
- **Benefits**: Promotes restful sleep and soothes postpartum fatigue.

30. Dried Fruit Mix for Energy

- **Ingredients**: 1/4 cup dried figs, 1/4 cup dried apricots, 1/4 cup raisins.
- **Method**: Combine dried fruits and snack on them throughout the day.
- **Benefits**: Provides iron, fiber, and sustained energy.

Menopause and Aging

1. Sage Tea for Hot Flashes

- **Ingredients**: 1 tsp dried sage leaves, 1 cup boiling water.
- **Method**: Steep sage in boiling water for 10 minutes. Strain and sip.
- **Benefits**: Reduces the frequency and intensity of hot flashes.

2. Flaxseed Water for Hormonal Balance

- **Ingredients**: 1 tbsp ground flaxseeds, 1 cup water.
- **Method**: Stir flaxseeds into water and drink daily.
- **Benefits**: Balances estrogen levels and eases menopausal symptoms.

3. Black Cohosh Tea for Night Sweats

- **Ingredients**: 1 tsp dried black cohosh root, 1 cup boiling water.
- **Method**: Steep black cohosh root in boiling water for 10 minutes. Strain and sip.
- **Benefits**: Reduces night sweats and supports hormonal regulation.

4. Ashwagandha Milk for Stress

- **Ingredients**: 1/2 tsp ashwagandha powder, 1 cup warm milk, 1 tsp honey.
- **Method**: Mix ashwagandha into milk, sweeten with honey, and drink before bed.
- **Benefits**: Reduces anxiety, improves sleep, and balances hormones.

5. Soy Milk for Hormonal Health

- **Ingredients**: 1 cup unsweetened soy milk.
- **Method**: Drink 1 cup of soy milk daily with breakfast.
- **Benefits**: Contains phytoestrogens that mimic estrogen to alleviate menopause symptoms.

6. Chamomile Tea for Mood Swings

- **Ingredients**: 1 tsp dried chamomile flowers, 1 cup boiling water.
- **Method**: Steep chamomile in boiling water for 10 minutes. Strain and drink before bed.
- **Benefits**: Calms the mind, reduces mood swings, and promotes restful sleep.

7. Red Clover Tea for Hot Flashes

- **Ingredients**: 1 tsp dried red clover flowers, 1 cup boiling water.
- **Method**: Steep red clover in boiling water for 10 minutes. Strain and sip.
- **Benefits**: Reduces hot flashes and improves bone health.

8. Vitamin E Oil Massage for Skin Elasticity

- **Ingredients**: 2 tbsp vitamin E oil.
- **Method**: Massage vitamin E oil onto the face and neck every night before bed.
- **Benefits**: Improves skin elasticity and reduces fine lines.

9. Holy Basil Tea for Emotional Balance

- **Ingredients**: 1 tsp dried holy basil leaves, 1 cup boiling water.
- **Method**: Steep holy basil in boiling water for 10 minutes. Strain and drink daily.

- **Benefits**: Reduces anxiety and promotes emotional stability.

10. Cooling Peppermint Spray for Hot Flashes

- **Ingredients**: 1 cup distilled water, 5 drops peppermint essential oil, a spray bottle.
- **Method**: Mix water and peppermint oil in a spray bottle. Mist onto the face and neck during hot flashes.
- **Benefits**: Provides instant cooling and relief.

11. Sesame Seed Snack for Bone Health

- **Ingredients**: 1 tbsp sesame seeds.
- **Method**: Eat 1 tbsp of sesame seeds daily as a snack or add to salads.
- **Benefits**: Rich in calcium to strengthen bones.

12. Lavender Diffusion for Better Sleep

- **Ingredients**: 4 drops lavender essential oil, a diffuser, water.
- **Method**: Add lavender oil to a diffuser with water and run it in your bedroom before sleep.
- **Benefits**: Promotes deep relaxation and reduces insomnia.

13. Turmeric Tea for Joint Health

- **Ingredients**: 1/2 tsp turmeric powder, 1 cup warm water, a pinch of black pepper.
- **Method**: Mix turmeric and black pepper into warm water and sip.
- **Benefits**: Reduces inflammation and supports joint health.

14. Dandelion Root Tea for Detox

- **Ingredients**: 1 tsp dried dandelion root, 1 cup boiling water.
- **Method**: Simmer dandelion root in boiling water for 10 minutes. Strain and drink.
- **Benefits**: Supports liver health and detoxifies the body.

15. Fenugreek Water for Libido

- **Ingredients**: 1 tsp fenugreek seeds, 1 cup water.
- **Method**: Soak fenugreek seeds in water overnight, strain, and drink in the morning.
- **Benefits**: Improves libido and balances hormones.

16. Coconut Oil Massage for Vaginal Dryness

- **Ingredients**: 1 tsp organic coconut oil.
- **Method**: Apply coconut oil gently to the vaginal area as needed.
- **Benefits**: Moisturizes and soothes dryness naturally.

17. Oatmeal Mask for Aging Skin

- **Ingredients**: 2 tbsp oats, 1 tsp honey, 1 tsp yogurt.
- **Method**: Mix into a paste, apply to the face, leave for 15 minutes, and rinse.
- **Benefits**: Exfoliates, hydrates, and rejuvenates aging skin.

18. Rosemary Tea for Mental Clarity

- **Ingredients**: 1 tsp dried rosemary leaves, 1 cup boiling water.
- **Method**: Steep rosemary in boiling water for 10 minutes. Strain and drink.
- **Benefits**: Enhances memory and mental clarity.

19. Evening Primrose Oil Capsules for Hormonal Balance

- **Ingredients**: 1 evening primrose oil capsule (consult dosage on label).
- **Method**: Take 1 capsule daily with food.
- **Benefits**: Eases hot flashes, mood swings, and breast tenderness.

20. Almond and Date Smoothie for Energy

- **Ingredients**: 1/4 cup almonds, 2 dates, 1 cup almond milk.
- **Method**: Blend all ingredients into a smoothie and drink.
- **Benefits**: Boosts energy and provides essential nutrients.

21. Epsom Salt Bath for Muscle Aches

- **Ingredients**: 1 cup Epsom salt, warm bathwater.
- **Method**: Dissolve salt in the bath and soak for 20 minutes.
- **Benefits**: Reduces muscle tension and promotes relaxation.

22. Cardamom Milk for Hormonal Health

- **Ingredients**: 1/4 tsp cardamom powder, 1 cup warm milk.
- **Method**: Mix cardamom into warm milk and drink before bed.

- **Benefits**: Supports hormonal balance and promotes restful sleep.

23. Aloe Vera Gel for Cooling Relief

- **Ingredients**: 2 tbsp fresh aloe vera gel.
- **Method**: Apply aloe vera gel to the chest and face to soothe hot flashes.
- **Benefits**: Provides instant cooling and hydrates the skin.

24. Beetroot Juice for Blood Flow

- **Ingredients**: 1/2 cup beetroot juice, 1/2 cup water.
- **Method**: Blend beetroot with water, strain, and drink.
- **Benefits**: Improves circulation and reduces fatigue.

25. Coriander Seed Water for Inflammation

- **Ingredients**: 1 tsp coriander seeds, 1 cup boiling water.
- **Method**: Simmer coriander seeds in boiling water for 10 minutes. Strain and sip.
- **Benefits**: Reduces inflammation and supports digestion.

26. Mint and Cucumber Infusion for Hydration

- **Ingredients**: 1/2 cucumber (sliced), 5 mint leaves, 1 liter water.
- **Method**: Infuse mint and cucumber in water for 1 hour and sip throughout the day.
- **Benefits**: Hydrates and cools the body.

27. Licorice Root Tea for Hormonal Support

- **Ingredients**: 1/2 tsp dried licorice root, 1 cup boiling water.
- **Method**: Steep licorice root in boiling water for 10 minutes. Strain and sip.
- **Benefits**: Supports adrenal health and balances hormones.

28. Papaya Salad for Digestion and Skin Health

- **Ingredients**: 1/2 cup ripe papaya, 1 tbsp lime juice, a pinch of salt.
- **Method**: Toss papaya with lime juice and salt. Eat fresh.
- **Benefits**: Improves digestion and supports glowing skin.

29. Probiotic Yogurt for Gut and Hormonal Health

- **Ingredients**: 1 cup plain probiotic yogurt.
- **Method**: Eat yogurt as a daily snack or with meals.
- **Benefits**: Balances gut bacteria, improving digestion and hormone regulation.

30. Lemon Balm Compress for Tension

- **Ingredients**: 1 tsp dried lemon balm, a clean cloth, 1 cup boiling water.
- **Method**: Steep lemon balm in boiling water, soak the cloth, and apply to the temples or neck.
- **Benefits**: Relieves headaches and calms tension.

3.6 Children's Remedies

Colds and Fevers

1. Chamomile Tea for Fever Relief

- **Ingredients**: 1 tsp dried chamomile flowers, 1 cup warm water.
- **Method**: Steep chamomile in warm water for 5–7 minutes, strain, and let cool. Give 1–2 tsp to younger children or 1/4 cup to older children.
- **Benefits**: Calms restlessness, reduces mild fever, and soothes the child.

2. Warm Lemon and Honey Drink for Sore Throat

- **Ingredients**: Juice of 1/2 lemon, 1 tsp honey, 1 cup warm water.
- **Method**: Mix ingredients and let your child sip slowly. (Not for children under 1 year old due to honey.)
- **Benefits**: Eases throat irritation and supports hydration.

3. Basil Tea for Colds

- **Ingredients**: 5 fresh basil leaves, 1 cup boiling water.
- **Method**: Steep basil leaves in water for 5 minutes, strain, and let cool before serving in small sips.
- **Benefits**: Helps reduce cold symptoms and supports immune health.

4. Onion Steam for Nasal Congestion

- **Ingredients**: 1 small onion (sliced), bowl of hot water.
- **Method**: Place onion slices in a bowl of hot water, have your child inhale the steam (supervised).
- **Benefits**: Opens up stuffy noses and reduces sinus congestion.

5. Cinnamon and Honey Paste for Cough Relief

- **Ingredients**: 1/4 tsp cinnamon powder, 1 tsp honey.
- **Method**: Mix into a paste and give 1/2 tsp to children over 1 year old.
- **Benefits**: Soothes coughs and provides antimicrobial properties.

6. Warm Compress for Fever

- **Ingredients**: A clean cloth, warm water.
- **Method**: Soak the cloth in warm water, wring out excess, and place on the child's forehead or back.
- **Benefits**: Gently reduces fever and provides comfort.

7. Ginger Bath for Body Aches

- **Ingredients**: 1 tsp grated ginger, warm bathwater.
- **Method**: Add grated ginger to the bathwater and let your child soak for 10–15 minutes.
- **Benefits**: Eases muscle aches and promotes sweating for fever reduction.

8. Honey and Clove Syrup for Sore Throats

- **Ingredients**: 1/2 tsp clove powder, 2 tbsp honey.
- **Method**: Mix ingredients and give 1/4 tsp to children over 1 year old.
- **Benefits**: Soothes sore throats and has mild antibacterial effects.

9. Dill Seed Tea for Congestion

- **Ingredients**: 1/2 tsp dill seeds, 1 cup water.
- **Method**: Simmer dill seeds in water for 5 minutes, strain, and cool before offering 1–2 tsp.
- **Benefits**: Relieves mild congestion and supports digestion.

10. Eucalyptus Chest Rub for Cough Relief

- **Ingredients**: 2 drops eucalyptus essential oil, 1 tbsp coconut oil.
- **Method**: Mix and rub gently on the child's chest before bedtime (for kids over 2 years old).
- **Benefits**: Opens airways and reduces coughing.

11. Warm Apple Juice for Hydration During Fever

- **Ingredients**: 1/2 cup warm, unsweetened apple juice.
- **Method**: Warm the juice slightly and give to the child in small sips.
- **Benefits**: Keeps the child hydrated and provides a soothing, mild flavor.

12. Carrot Soup for Immune Support

- **Ingredients**: 1/2 cup chopped carrots, 1 cup water, a pinch of salt.
- **Method**: Simmer carrots until soft, blend into a soup, and serve warm.
- **Benefits**: Nourishes the body and supports immune health during a cold.

13. Peppermint Steam for Stuffy Noses

- **Ingredients**: 1 drop peppermint essential oil, bowl of hot water.
- **Method**: Add oil to hot water and let the child inhale the steam (supervised).
- **Benefits**: Clears nasal passages and reduces congestion.

14. Herbal Foot Soak for Cold Relief

- **Ingredients**: 1 tsp dried rosemary, 1 tsp dried thyme, warm water.
- **Method**: Add herbs to a basin of warm water, soak your child's feet for 10 minutes.
- **Benefits**: Stimulates circulation and soothes cold symptoms.

15. Honey and Ginger Drink for Fever and Cough

- **Ingredients**: 1/2 tsp grated ginger, 1 tsp honey, 1 cup warm water.
- **Method**: Mix ingredients and give in small sips to children over 1 year old.
- **Benefits**: Reduces fever and soothes coughs.

16. Tulsi and Mint Tea for Colds

- **Ingredients**: 5 fresh tulsi leaves, 5 fresh mint leaves, 1 cup boiling water.
- **Method**: Steep leaves in boiling water for 5 minutes, strain, and cool. Give in small sips.
- **Benefits**: Combines antiviral and soothing properties for cold relief.

17. Aloe Vera Gel for Soothing Fevers

- **Ingredients**: 2 tbsp fresh aloe vera gel.
- **Method**: Apply a thin layer of aloe vera gel to the child's forehead or chest.
- **Benefits**: Provides cooling relief for feverish discomfort.

18. Cinnamon Milk for Coughs

- **Ingredients**: 1 cup warm milk, 1/4 tsp cinnamon powder.
- **Method**: Mix cinnamon into milk and let the child drink before bed.
- **Benefits**: Reduces coughing and supports restful sleep.

19. Lemon and Salt Compress for Fevers

- **Ingredients**: 1/2 lemon (sliced), a clean cloth, warm water.

- **Method**: Soak the cloth in warm water with lemon slices and place it on the child's feet or forehead.
- **Benefits**: Gently reduces fever and refreshes.

20. Clove Tea for Sore Throats

- **Ingredients**: 2 cloves, 1 cup water.
- **Method**: Simmer cloves in water for 5 minutes, strain, and cool before serving in small sips.
- **Benefits**: Soothes sore throats and reduces inflammation.

21. Turmeric Milk for Mild Fevers

- **Ingredients**: 1 cup warm milk, 1/4 tsp turmeric powder.
- **Method**: Mix turmeric into milk and let the child sip slowly.
- **Benefits**: Reduces mild fever and strengthens immunity.

22. Caraway Seed Tea for Runny Nose

- **Ingredients**: 1/2 tsp caraway seeds, 1 cup water.
- **Method**: Simmer seeds in water for 5 minutes, strain, and cool.
- **Benefits**: Reduces runny nose and supports respiratory health.

23. Warm Ginger Compress for Chest Congestion

- **Ingredients**: 1 tsp grated ginger, warm water, a clean cloth.
- **Method**: Soak the cloth in ginger-infused warm water, wring out, and place on the chest.
- **Benefits**: Loosens mucus and eases breathing.

24. Mashed Banana with Honey for Cough Relief

- **Ingredients**: 1 ripe banana, 1 tsp honey.
- **Method**: Mash banana with honey and give 1–2 tsp to older children.
- **Benefits**: Soothes the throat and suppresses coughing.

25. Thyme Steam for Sinus Relief

- **Ingredients**: 1 tsp dried thyme, bowl of hot water.
- **Method**: Add thyme to hot water, let the child inhale the steam (supervised).
- **Benefits**: Clears sinuses and reduces congestion.

26. Mint Oil Rub for Colds

- **Ingredients**: 2 drops mint essential oil, 1 tsp coconut oil.
- **Method**: Mix oils and massage onto the chest or back.
- **Benefits**: Opens airways and reduces cold symptoms.

27. Dill Seed Compress for Feverish Discomfort

- **Ingredients**: 1 tsp dill seeds, warm water, a clean cloth.
- **Method**: Soak the cloth in dill-infused water and place it on the forehead.
- **Benefits**: Soothes mild fever and provides comfort.

28. Cucumber and Aloe Smoothie for Hydration

- **Ingredients**: 1/2 cucumber, 2 tbsp aloe vera gel, 1/4 cup water.
- **Method**: Blend and serve in small portions.
- **Benefits**: Hydrates and cools feverish children.

29. Anise Seed Tea for Colds

- **Ingredients**: 1/2 tsp anise seeds, 1 cup boiling water.
- **Method**: Steep seeds in boiling water for 5 minutes, strain, and cool.
- **Benefits**: Relieves congestion and soothes coughing.

30. Restorative Broth for Recovery

- **Ingredients**: 1/2 cup chopped carrots, celery, and onions, 2 cups water.
- **Method**: Simmer vegetables in water for 20 minutes, strain, and serve warm.
- **Benefits**: Provides nutrients to aid recovery and hydration.

Tummy Troubles

1. Dill Seed Tea for Infant Colic

- **Ingredients**: 1/2 tsp dill seeds, 1 cup water.
- **Method**: Simmer dill seeds in water for 5 minutes, strain, and cool. Give 1–2 tsp to infants or 1/4 cup to older children.
- **Benefits**: Relieves gas and soothes colicky pain.

2. Fennel Seed Tea for Gas Relief

- **Ingredients**: 1/2 tsp fennel seeds, 1 cup water.
- **Method**: Steep fennel seeds in boiling water for 10 minutes, strain, and cool. Give in small sips.
- **Benefits**: Eases gas and bloating.

3. Warm Compress for Stomach Pain

- **Ingredients**: A clean cloth, warm water.
- **Method**: Soak the cloth in warm water, wring out excess, and place on the child's tummy.
- **Benefits**: Relieves cramps and provides comfort.

4. Ginger Water for Nausea

- **Ingredients**: 1/4 tsp grated ginger, 1 cup water.
- **Method**: Boil ginger in water for 5 minutes, strain, and cool. Offer 1–2 tsp to children over 1 year old.
- **Benefits**: Reduces nausea and eases digestion.

5. Mint and Honey Drink for Indigestion

- **Ingredients**: 1 tsp fresh mint leaves, 1 tsp honey, 1 cup warm water.
- **Method**: Steep mint leaves in warm water for 5 minutes, strain, and add honey.
- **Benefits**: Relieves indigestion and soothes upset tummies.

6. Caraway Seed Tea for Colicky Babies

- **Ingredients**: 1/2 tsp caraway seeds, 1 cup water.
- **Method**: Simmer caraway seeds in water for 5 minutes, strain, and let cool. Give in small sips.
- **Benefits**: Reduces gas and soothes colicky pain.

7. Chamomile Tea for Relaxation and Digestion

- **Ingredients**: 1 tsp dried chamomile flowers, 1 cup boiling water.
- **Method**: Steep chamomile in boiling water for 5–7 minutes, strain, and let cool.
- **Benefits**: Calms tummy discomfort and relaxes the child.

8. Lemon Water for Mild Nausea

- **Ingredients**: Juice of 1/2 lemon, 1 cup water.
- **Method**: Mix lemon juice with water and let the child sip slowly.
- **Benefits**: Soothes nausea and supports hydration.

9. Yogurt for Gut Health

- **Ingredients**: 1/4 cup plain probiotic yogurt.
- **Method**: Serve plain or mix with a bit of honey for children over 1 year old.
- **Benefits**: Promotes healthy digestion and eases diarrhea.

10. Cumin Seed Water for Gas

- **Ingredients**: 1/2 tsp cumin seeds, 1 cup water.
- **Method**: Simmer cumin seeds in water for 5 minutes, strain, and cool.
- **Benefits**: Reduces bloating and gas.

11. Peppermint Tea for Stomach Cramps

- **Ingredients**: 1 tsp dried peppermint leaves, 1 cup boiling water.
- **Method**: Steep peppermint leaves in boiling water for 10 minutes, strain, and cool.
- **Benefits**: Relaxes stomach muscles and eases cramps.

12. Banana and Honey Mash for Diarrhea

- **Ingredients**: 1 ripe banana, 1 tsp honey.
- **Method**: Mash the banana with honey and serve.
- **Benefits**: Binds loose stools and restores energy.

13. Warm Rice Water for Upset Stomach

- **Ingredients**: 1/2 cup rice, 2 cups water.
- **Method**: Boil rice in water, strain the liquid, and let cool. Offer in small sips.
- **Benefits**: Soothes the stomach and prevents dehydration.

14. Apple Sauce for Diarrhea

- **Ingredients**: 1/2 cup unsweetened applesauce.
- **Method**: Serve chilled.
- **Benefits**: Eases diarrhea and provides nutrients.

15. Baking Soda Drink for Heartburn

- **Ingredients**: 1/4 tsp baking soda, 1 cup water.
- **Method**: Dissolve baking soda in water and give small sips.
- **Benefits**: Neutralizes acidity and relieves heartburn.

16. Dill and Honey Drops for Gas

- **Ingredients**: 1/2 tsp dill seeds, 1 tsp honey.
- **Method**: Crush dill seeds and mix with honey. Offer small drops to children over 1 year old.
- **Benefits**: Eases gas and soothes tummy pain.

17. Clove Tea for Stomach Infections

- **Ingredients**: 2 cloves, 1 cup boiling water.
- **Method**: Simmer cloves in water for 5 minutes, strain, and cool.
- **Benefits**: Antimicrobial properties soothe stomach infections.

18. Buttermilk with Cumin for Digestive Health

- **Ingredients**: 1/4 cup plain buttermilk, a pinch of cumin powder.
- **Method**: Mix cumin into buttermilk and serve chilled.
- **Benefits**: Eases bloating and improves digestion.

19. Papaya Puree for Constipation

- **Ingredients**: 1/4 cup ripe papaya.
- **Method**: Mash papaya into a smooth puree and serve.
- **Benefits**: Relieves constipation and supports digestion.

20. Anise Seed Tea for Colic

- **Ingredients**: 1/2 tsp anise seeds, 1 cup water.
- **Method**: Simmer seeds in water for 5 minutes, strain, and cool.
- **Benefits**: Reduces colic and gas.

21. Warm Milk with Turmeric for Gas

- **Ingredients**: 1 cup warm milk, 1/4 tsp turmeric powder.

- **Method**: Mix turmeric into warm milk and give in small sips.
- **Benefits**: Relieves gas and bloating.

22. Carrot Soup for Recovery

- **Ingredients**: 1/2 cup chopped carrots, 1 cup water, a pinch of salt.
- **Method**: Boil carrots until soft, blend into a soup, and serve warm.
- **Benefits**: Eases digestion and nourishes the body.

23. Pomegranate Juice for Upset Stomach

- **Ingredients**: 1/2 cup fresh pomegranate juice.
- **Method**: Serve fresh in small sips.
- **Benefits**: Soothes the stomach and reduces nausea.

24. Aloe Vera Juice for Constipation

- **Ingredients**: 1 tbsp fresh aloe vera gel, 1/4 cup water.
- **Method**: Blend aloe vera gel with water and serve small portions.
- **Benefits**: Gently relieves constipation.

25. Raisin Water for Constipation

- **Ingredients**: 5 raisins, 1/2 cup water.
- **Method**: Soak raisins overnight, mash, and strain the water. Offer in small sips.
- **Benefits**: Eases constipation naturally.

26. Cardamom and Ginger Drink for Nausea

- **Ingredients**: 1 cardamom pod, 1/4 tsp grated ginger, 1 cup water.
- **Method**: Simmer cardamom and ginger in water for 5 minutes, strain, and cool.
- **Benefits**: Combats nausea and soothes digestion.

27. Basil Leaf Infusion for Tummy Ache

- **Ingredients**: 3 fresh basil leaves, 1 cup boiling water.
- **Method**: Steep basil leaves in boiling water for 5 minutes, strain, and cool.
- **Benefits**: Relieves tummy pain and improves digestion.

28. Coconut Water for Dehydration

- **Ingredients**: 1/2 cup fresh coconut water.
- **Method**: Serve chilled in small sips.
- **Benefits**: Rehydrates and soothes upset stomachs.

29. Honey and Cinnamon Drink for Cramps

- **Ingredients**: 1/4 tsp cinnamon powder, 1 tsp honey, 1 cup warm water.
- **Method**: Mix and give in small sips to children over 1 year old.
- **Benefits**: Relieves cramps and reduces inflammation.

30. Plain Toast for Nausea

- **Ingredients**: 1 slice of plain toast.
- **Method**: Toast bread lightly and serve plain.
- **Benefits**: Settles nausea and absorbs stomach acids.

Sleep and Stress

1. Warm Milk with Honey for Relaxation

- **Ingredients**: 1 cup warm milk, 1 tsp honey.
- **Method**: Mix honey into warm milk and give to the child 30 minutes before bed.
- **Benefits**: Encourages relaxation and helps the child fall asleep easily.

2. Lavender Pillow Spray for Sleep

- **Ingredients**: 1/2 cup distilled water, 5 drops lavender essential oil, spray bottle.
- **Method**: Mix water and lavender oil in a spray bottle. Lightly mist the child's pillow before bedtime.
- **Benefits**: Promotes calmness and relaxation.

3. Chamomile Tea for Bedtime Calm

- **Ingredients**: 1 tsp dried chamomile flowers, 1 cup warm water.
- **Method**: Steep chamomile flowers in warm water for 5–7 minutes, strain, and cool slightly.
- **Benefits**: Reduces restlessness and helps induce sleep.

4. Lavender and Coconut Oil Massage for Stress Relief

- **Ingredients**: 1 drop lavender essential oil, 1 tbsp coconut oil.
- **Method**: Mix oils and gently massage the child's back or feet before bed.
- **Benefits**: Relaxes tense muscles and calms the mind.

5. Epsom Salt Bath for Relaxation

- **Ingredients**: 1/2 cup Epsom salt, warm bathwater.
- **Method**: Dissolve Epsom salt in warm water and let the child soak for 15 minutes.
- **Benefits**: Eases muscle tension and promotes better sleep.

6. Warm Compress for Soothing Restlessness

- **Ingredients**: A clean cloth, warm water.
- **Method**: Soak the cloth in warm water, wring it out, and place on the child's forehead or feet.
- **Benefits**: Provides comfort and helps calm a restless child.

7. Lemon Balm Tea for Anxiety

- **Ingredients**: 1 tsp dried lemon balm, 1 cup warm water.
- **Method**: Steep lemon balm in warm water for 5 minutes, strain, and let the child sip slowly.
- **Benefits**: Reduces mild anxiety and promotes emotional balance.

8. Soft Music Therapy for Sleep

- **Ingredients**: None.
- **Method**: Play soothing, gentle music during bedtime to create a relaxing environment.
- **Benefits**: Helps calm the mind and eases the child into sleep.

9. Jasmine Oil Diffusion for Emotional Calm

- **Ingredients**: 3 drops jasmine essential oil, water, diffuser.
- **Method**: Add jasmine oil and water to a diffuser and run it in the bedroom for 30 minutes before bedtime.
- **Benefits**: Reduces stress and encourages a sense of security.

10. Banana and Almond Smoothie for Better Sleep

- **Ingredients**: 1/2 banana, 1 tsp almond butter, 1/2 cup milk.

- **Method**: Blend ingredients into a smooth drink and serve before bed.
- **Benefits**: Contains magnesium and tryptophan, which help promote sleep.

11. Mint Tea for Overactive Minds

- **Ingredients**: 1 tsp dried mint leaves, 1 cup warm water.
- **Method**: Steep mint leaves in warm water for 5–7 minutes, strain, and cool slightly.
- **Benefits**: Calms the mind and reduces overstimulation.

12. Stuffed Animal Lavender Sachets for Comfort

- **Ingredients**: Dried lavender flowers, a small cloth pouch.
- **Method**: Fill the pouch with lavender flowers and tuck it inside the child's stuffed animal or place it near the pillow.
- **Benefits**: Provides a calming scent to ease anxiety and help the child sleep.

13. Warm Oatmeal Snack for Sleep

- **Ingredients**: 1/4 cup oats, 1/2 cup milk, 1 tsp honey.
- **Method**: Cook oats with milk, stir in honey, and serve warm before bedtime.
- **Benefits**: Stabilizes blood sugar and promotes a sense of comfort.

14. Bedtime Story for Emotional Soothing

- **Ingredients**: A gentle, calming book.
- **Method**: Read a soothing bedtime story in a quiet, relaxed tone before sleep.
- **Benefits**: Helps the child transition into a peaceful state of mind.

15. Rose Oil Massage for Emotional Calm

- **Ingredients**: 1 drop rose essential oil, 1 tsp carrier oil (e.g., coconut oil).
- **Method**: Mix oils and gently massage the child's hands or feet.
- **Benefits**: Reduces anxiety and promotes emotional well-being.

16. Cardamom Milk for Stress Relief

- **Ingredients**: 1 cup warm milk, 1/4 tsp cardamom powder.
- **Method**: Mix cardamom into warm milk and give to the child before bed.
- **Benefits**: Soothes restlessness and encourages relaxation.

17. Deep Breathing Practice for Anxiety

- **Ingredients**: None.
- **Method**: Teach the child to inhale deeply through the nose, hold for 3 seconds, and exhale slowly through the mouth. Repeat 5 times.
- **Benefits**: Calms the nervous system and reduces anxiety.

18. Warm Apple Cider Drink for Comfort

- **Ingredients**: 1/2 cup warm apple cider, a pinch of cinnamon.
- **Method**: Warm the cider, sprinkle with cinnamon, and serve before bedtime.
- **Benefits**: Provides a cozy, calming effect for better sleep.

19. Lavender Bath Bomb for Relaxation

- **Ingredients**: 1/2 cup baking soda, 1/4 cup citric acid, 5 drops lavender essential oil.
- **Method**: Mix ingredients, shape into balls, and let dry. Use in a warm bath.
- **Benefits**: Creates a calming and soothing bath experience.

20. Basil Tea for Emotional Stability

- **Ingredients**: 3 fresh basil leaves, 1 cup warm water.
- **Method**: Steep basil leaves in warm water for 5 minutes, strain, and cool slightly.
- **Benefits**: Eases stress and improves mood.

21. Lavender and Rice Heat Pack for Comfort

- **Ingredients**: 1/2 cup dried rice, 2 tbsp dried lavender flowers, a clean sock.
- **Method**: Fill the sock with rice and lavender, tie it closed, and microwave for 30 seconds. Use as a warm pack.
- **Benefits**: Provides warmth and a calming scent to ease tension.

22. Honey and Cinnamon Drink for Restless Nights

- **Ingredients**: 1 tsp honey, a pinch of cinnamon, 1 cup warm water.
- **Method**: Mix ingredients and serve in small sips.
- **Benefits**: Soothes and relaxes the body for better sleep.

23. Orange Peel Pillow Sachet for Relaxation

- **Ingredients**: Dried orange peels, a small pouch.
- **Method**: Fill the pouch with dried orange peels and tuck it near the child's pillow.
- **Benefits**: Provides a mild citrus scent that promotes relaxation.

24. Coconut Water for Bedtime Hydration

- **Ingredients**: 1/4 cup fresh coconut water.
- **Method**: Serve chilled coconut water before bedtime.
- **Benefits**: Hydrates and soothes the child.

25. Vanilla Milk for Emotional Comfort

- **Ingredients**: 1 cup warm milk, 1/4 tsp vanilla extract.
- **Method**: Stir vanilla into milk and serve.
- **Benefits**: Calms nerves and promotes emotional comfort.

26. Lavender and Chamomile Sachet for Sleep

- **Ingredients**: Dried lavender and chamomile flowers, a small cloth pouch.
- **Method**: Fill the pouch with the flowers and place it near the child's bed.
- **Benefits**: Combines calming scents to promote deep sleep.

27. Soft Night Light for Security

- **Ingredients**: A soft, dim night light.
- **Method**: Place the night light in the child's room to create a comforting environment.
- **Benefits**: Reduces nighttime anxiety and promotes a sense of safety.

28. Ginger Tea for Stress-Induced Tummy Aches

- **Ingredients**: 1/4 tsp grated ginger, 1 cup warm water.
- **Method**: Simmer ginger in water for 5 minutes, strain, and let cool slightly.
- **Benefits**: Soothes stress-related stomach discomfort.

29. Lavender and Mint Steam Inhalation for Calmness

- **Ingredients**: 1 drop lavender oil, 1 drop mint oil, bowl of hot water.
- **Method**: Add oils to hot water and let the child inhale the steam under supervision.
- **Benefits**: Clears the mind and promotes relaxation.

30. Deep Hug Therapy for Emotional Security

- **Ingredients**: None.
- **Method**: Give the child a warm, gentle hug for a few moments before bed.
- **Benefits**: Instills a sense of safety, reduces stress, and strengthens the bond.

3.7 First Aid and Emergency Remedies

Cuts, Scrapes, and Wounds

1. Plantain Poultice for Wound Healing

- **Ingredients**: 5 fresh plantain leaves, a mortar and pestle.
- **Method**: Crush the leaves into a paste and apply directly to the wound. Cover with a clean cloth or bandage.
- **Benefits**: Antimicrobial and anti-inflammatory properties promote healing.

2. Honey Dressing for Preventing Infection

- **Ingredients**: 1 tsp raw honey, a clean bandage.
- **Method**: Spread a thin layer of honey on the wound and cover with a bandage. Change daily.
- **Benefits**: Acts as a natural antibiotic and prevents infections.

3. Turmeric Paste for Antibacterial Action

- **Ingredients**: 1/2 tsp turmeric powder, a few drops of water.
- **Method**: Mix into a paste, apply to the wound, and cover with a bandage.
- **Benefits**: Fights bacteria and speeds up healing.

4. Aloe Vera Gel for Soothing Cuts

- **Ingredients**: 2 tbsp fresh aloe vera gel.
- **Method**: Apply the gel directly to the wound and let it dry. Repeat 2–3 times daily.
- **Benefits**: Soothes the skin and accelerates tissue repair.

5. Calendula Salve for Healing

- **Ingredients**: 1/4 cup calendula-infused oil, 1 tbsp beeswax.
- **Method**: Melt beeswax, mix with calendula oil, and cool. Apply to wounds as needed.
- **Benefits**: Reduces inflammation and encourages new tissue growth.

6. Garlic Compress for Infection Prevention

- **Ingredients**: 1 clove garlic (crushed), a clean cloth.
- **Method**: Wrap crushed garlic in the cloth, place it on the wound for 5–10 minutes, and then remove.
- **Benefits**: Natural antibacterial properties fight infections.

7. Lavender Essential Oil for Disinfecting

- **Ingredients**: 2 drops lavender essential oil, 1 tsp coconut oil.
- **Method**: Mix and apply to the wound with a cotton swab.
- **Benefits**: Disinfects the wound and promotes relaxation.

8. Witch Hazel for Reducing Swelling

- **Ingredients**: 1 tsp witch hazel.
- **Method**: Dab witch hazel on the wound using a cotton ball.
- **Benefits**: Reduces swelling and prevents infection.

9. Tea Tree Oil Ointment for Cuts

- **Ingredients**: 1 drop tea tree oil, 1 tsp olive oil.
- **Method**: Mix oils and apply to the wound with a clean cotton swab.
- **Benefits**: Fights bacteria and reduces inflammation.

10. Comfrey Poultice for Tissue Regeneration

- **Ingredients**: 1 tbsp comfrey leaves, a mortar and pestle.
- **Method**: Crush the leaves into a paste and apply to the wound. Cover with a bandage.
- **Benefits**: Encourages tissue regeneration and speeds healing.

11. Chamomile Tea Rinse for Gentle Cleaning

- **Ingredients**: 1 chamomile tea bag, 1 cup boiling water.
- **Method**: Steep the tea bag, let it cool, and use the liquid to rinse the wound.
- **Benefits**: Cleanses and soothes the skin while reducing inflammation.

12. Coconut Oil for Moisturizing Wounds

- **Ingredients**: 1 tsp virgin coconut oil.
- **Method**: Apply directly to the wound and cover with a bandage.

- **Benefits**: Keeps the wound moist and prevents scarring.

13. Goldenseal Powder for Infection Control

- **Ingredients**: 1/2 tsp goldenseal powder, a few drops of water.
- **Method**: Mix into a paste and apply to the wound. Cover with a bandage.
- **Benefits**: Natural antibiotic properties prevent infection.

14. Basil Juice for Antimicrobial Protection

- **Ingredients**: 5 fresh basil leaves.
- **Method**: Crush the leaves to extract juice and apply directly to the wound.
- **Benefits**: Fights bacteria and supports healing.

15. Echinacea Tea Wash for Immune Support

- **Ingredients**: 1 tsp dried echinacea, 1 cup boiling water.
- **Method**: Steep echinacea in boiling water, let it cool, and use as a wound wash.
- **Benefits**: Boosts local immunity and speeds recovery.

16. Thyme Infusion for Cleaning Cuts

- **Ingredients**: 1 tsp dried thyme, 1 cup boiling water.
- **Method**: Steep thyme in boiling water, let it cool, and rinse the wound with the liquid.
- **Benefits**: Antiseptic properties clean the wound and reduce infection risk.

17. Raw Potato Poultice for Drawing Out Infection

- **Ingredients**: 1 raw potato (grated).
- **Method**: Place the grated potato on the wound, cover with a cloth, and leave for 20 minutes.
- **Benefits**: Draws out toxins and reduces swelling.

18. Onion Paste for Antimicrobial Action

- **Ingredients**: 1 small onion (blended into a paste).
- **Method**: Apply the paste to the wound and cover with a bandage.
- **Benefits**: Fights bacteria and supports healing.

19. Marshmallow Root Poultice for Soothing Wounds

- **Ingredients**: 1 tbsp marshmallow root powder, a few drops of water.
- **Method**: Mix into a paste and apply to the wound. Cover with a clean cloth.
- **Benefits**: Soothes inflammation and protects the wound.

20. Hydrogen Peroxide Rinse for Cleaning

- **Ingredients**: 1 tsp hydrogen peroxide, 1 cup water.
- **Method**: Dilute peroxide with water and rinse the wound gently.
- **Benefits**: Cleans the wound and prevents bacterial growth.

21. Calendula and Lavender Oil Mix for Healing

- **Ingredients**: 1 tsp calendula oil, 1 drop lavender oil.
- **Method**: Mix oils and apply to the wound with a cotton swab.
- **Benefits**: Combines soothing and healing properties.

22. Banana Peel Bandage for Soothing Cuts

- **Ingredients**: 1 piece of banana peel.
- **Method**: Place the inside of the peel on the wound and secure with a bandage.
- **Benefits**: Reduces irritation and speeds up healing.

23. Alum Powder for Bleeding Control

- **Ingredients**: 1/4 tsp alum powder.
- **Method**: Sprinkle alum powder on the wound to stop bleeding.
- **Benefits**: Astringent properties help control bleeding.

24. Yarrow Poultice for Bleeding Wounds

- **Ingredients**: 1 tbsp fresh yarrow leaves.
- **Method**: Crush the leaves into a paste and apply to the wound.
- **Benefits**: Stops bleeding and promotes clotting.

25. Beetroot Paste for Promoting Clotting

- **Ingredients**: 1/2 beetroot (grated).
- **Method**: Apply the grated beetroot to the wound and cover with a cloth.
- **Benefits**: Encourages clotting and soothes the wound.

26. Black Tea Compress for Reducing Inflammation

- **Ingredients**: 1 black tea bag, 1 cup warm water.
- **Method**: Soak the tea bag in warm water and place it on the wound for 10 minutes.
- **Benefits**: Reduces swelling and soothes the area.

27. Slippery Elm Powder Paste for Healing

- **Ingredients**: 1 tbsp slippery elm powder, a few drops of water.
- **Method**: Mix into a paste and apply to the wound.
- **Benefits**: Protects the wound and accelerates healing.

28. Rosewater Rinse for Gentle Cleaning

- **Ingredients**: 1/4 cup rosewater.
- **Method**: Rinse the wound with rosewater to clean it.
- **Benefits**: Cleanses gently and soothes irritated skin.

29. Turmeric and Honey Mix for Deep Cuts

- **Ingredients**: 1/2 tsp turmeric powder, 1 tsp honey.
- **Method**: Mix into a paste and apply to the wound.
- **Benefits**: Combines antibacterial and healing properties.

30. Ice Compress for Reducing Pain

- **Ingredients**: Ice cubes, a clean cloth.
- **Method**: Wrap ice cubes in the cloth and place gently over the wound for 5 minutes.
- **Benefits**: Numbs pain and reduces inflammation.

Burns and Bites

1. Aloe Vera Gel for Cooling Burns

- **Ingredients**: 2 tbsp fresh aloe vera gel.
- **Method**: Apply the gel directly to the burn and let it dry. Reapply 2–3 times daily.
- **Benefits**: Provides instant cooling, reduces pain, and promotes healing.

2. Honey Dressing for Burns

- **Ingredients**: 1 tsp raw honey, a clean bandage.
- **Method**: Spread honey on the burn and cover with a bandage. Change daily.
- **Benefits**: Soothes burns, prevents infection, and speeds up healing.

3. Lavender Essential Oil for Burns

- **Ingredients**: 2 drops lavender essential oil, 1 tsp coconut oil.
- **Method**: Mix and gently apply to the burn. Repeat twice daily.
- **Benefits**: Reduces pain, speeds healing, and prevents scarring.

4. Baking Soda Paste for Bug Bite Itching

- **Ingredients**: 1 tbsp baking soda, a few drops of water.
- **Method**: Mix into a paste and apply to the bite. Leave for 10 minutes and rinse.
- **Benefits**: Relieves itching and reduces swelling.

5. Tea Bag Compress for Burns

- **Ingredients**: 1 black tea bag, 1/4 cup cool water.
- **Method**: Soak the tea bag in cool water and place it on the burn for 10 minutes.
- **Benefits**: Reduces inflammation and soothes pain.

6. Calendula Salve for Minor Burns

- **Ingredients**: 1/4 cup calendula-infused oil, 1 tbsp beeswax.
- **Method**: Melt beeswax, mix with calendula oil, and cool. Apply to burns as needed.
- **Benefits**: Soothes and speeds the healing of minor burns.

7. Ice Compress for Bites

- **Ingredients**: Ice cubes, a clean cloth.
- **Method**: Wrap ice cubes in the cloth and place on the bite for 5–10 minutes.
- **Benefits**: Reduces swelling and numbs itching or pain.

8. Banana Peel for Mosquito Bites

- **Ingredients**: 1 piece of banana peel.

- **Method**: Rub the inside of the peel on the bite for relief.
- **Benefits**: Soothes itching and reduces redness.

9. Cucumber Slice for Burns

- **Ingredients**: 1 slice of cucumber.
- **Method**: Place the cucumber slice directly on the burn and leave for 15 minutes.
- **Benefits**: Cools the burn and reduces swelling.

10. Coconut Oil for Healing Burns

- **Ingredients**: 1 tsp coconut oil.
- **Method**: Gently apply coconut oil to the burn once it has cooled. Repeat twice daily.
- **Benefits**: Prevents dryness and promotes healing.

11. Apple Cider Vinegar for Bug Bites

- **Ingredients**: 1 tsp apple cider vinegar, 1 cup water.
- **Method**: Dilute the vinegar with water and dab onto the bite with a cotton ball.
- **Benefits**: Relieves itching and reduces inflammation.

12. Potato Slices for Burns

- **Ingredients**: 1 raw potato (sliced).
- **Method**: Place a slice of potato on the burn and leave for 10 minutes.
- **Benefits**: Soothes the skin and reduces pain.

13. Witch Hazel for Insect Bites

- **Ingredients**: 1 tsp witch hazel.
- **Method**: Apply witch hazel to the bite with a cotton ball.
- **Benefits**: Reduces itching, swelling, and irritation.

14. Basil Juice for Antibacterial Protection

- **Ingredients**: 5 fresh basil leaves.
- **Method**: Crush the leaves to extract juice and apply directly to the bite.
- **Benefits**: Relieves itching and prevents infection.

15. Turmeric and Honey Paste for Burns

- **Ingredients**: 1/2 tsp turmeric powder, 1 tsp honey.
- **Method**: Mix into a paste and apply to the burn. Leave for 20 minutes, then rinse.
- **Benefits**: Combines antibacterial and anti-inflammatory properties.

16. Peppermint Oil for Bites

- **Ingredients**: 1 drop peppermint essential oil, 1 tsp carrier oil (e.g., olive oil).
- **Method**: Mix oils and dab onto the bite.
- **Benefits**: Provides a cooling effect and reduces itching.

17. Oatmeal Paste for Bite Itching

- **Ingredients**: 1 tbsp ground oatmeal, a few drops of water.
- **Method**: Mix into a paste and apply to the bite. Leave for 10 minutes and rinse.
- **Benefits**: Reduces itching and soothes the skin.

18. Chamomile Tea Rinse for Burns

- **Ingredients**: 1 chamomile tea bag, 1 cup cool water.
- **Method**: Steep tea bag in water, cool, and rinse the burn with the liquid.
- **Benefits**: Soothes inflammation and promotes healing.

19. Onion Juice for Bug Bites

- **Ingredients**: 1 small onion.
- **Method**: Crush the onion to extract juice and dab it onto the bite.
- **Benefits**: Relieves itching and reduces redness.

20. Aloe and Lavender Gel for Burns

- **Ingredients**: 2 tbsp aloe vera gel, 2 drops lavender essential oil.
- **Method**: Mix and apply directly to the burn.
- **Benefits**: Soothes and accelerates healing.

21. Papaya Pulp for Insect Bites

- **Ingredients**: 1 tbsp mashed papaya.
- **Method**: Apply pulp to the bite and leave for 15 minutes.

- **Benefits**: Reduces inflammation and itching.

22. Baking Soda and Honey Mix for Burns

- **Ingredients**: 1 tsp baking soda, 1 tsp honey.
- **Method**: Mix into a paste and apply to the burn. Leave for 20 minutes, then rinse.
- **Benefits**: Combines cooling and antimicrobial effects.

23. Garlic Paste for Bites

- **Ingredients**: 1 clove garlic (crushed).
- **Method**: Apply the paste to the bite, leave for 5 minutes, then rinse off.
- **Benefits**: Prevents infection and reduces swelling.

24. Tea Tree Oil for Bites and Stings

- **Ingredients**: 1 drop tea tree oil, 1 tsp coconut oil.
- **Method**: Mix and apply to the bite with a cotton swab.
- **Benefits**: Fights bacteria and reduces irritation.

25. Ice and Salt Compress for Bites

- **Ingredients**: Ice cubes, a pinch of salt, a clean cloth.
- **Method**: Wrap ice cubes in a cloth, sprinkle with salt, and apply to the bite.
- **Benefits**: Reduces swelling and itching.

26. Slippery Elm Paste for Burns

- **Ingredients**: 1 tsp slippery elm powder, a few drops of water.
- **Method**: Mix into a paste and apply to the burn.
- **Benefits**: Soothes the burn and promotes healing.

27. Mint and Basil Paste for Mosquito Bites

- **Ingredients**: 2 fresh mint leaves, 2 fresh basil leaves.
- **Method**: Crush into a paste and apply to the bite.
- **Benefits**: Provides cooling relief and reduces irritation.

28. Rosewater Spray for Minor Burns

- **Ingredients**: 1/4 cup rosewater, spray bottle.
- **Method**: Spray rosewater onto the burn 2–3 times daily.
- **Benefits**: Cools the burn and reduces inflammation.

29. Aloe and Honey Mix for Insect Bites

- **Ingredients**: 1 tbsp aloe vera gel, 1 tsp honey.
- **Method**: Mix and apply to the bite.
- **Benefits**: Reduces swelling and soothes itching.

30. Beetroot Slice for Burns

- **Ingredients**: 1 slice of beetroot.
- **Method**: Place the beetroot slice on the burn for 10 minutes.
- **Benefits**: Draws out heat and reduces redness.

Bruises and Sprains

1. Arnica Gel for Bruises

- **Ingredients**: Store-bought arnica gel.
- **Method**: Apply a thin layer of arnica gel to the bruised area 2–3 times daily.
- **Benefits**: Reduces swelling, minimizes discoloration, and speeds up healing.

2. Cold Compress for Immediate Swelling

- **Ingredients**: Ice cubes, a clean cloth.
- **Method**: Wrap ice cubes in a cloth and place on the bruised or sprained area for 10–15 minutes.
- **Benefits**: Reduces swelling and numbs pain.

3. Warm Compress for Older Bruises

- **Ingredients**: A clean cloth, warm water.
- **Method**: Soak the cloth in warm water, wring out excess, and apply to the bruise for 10 minutes.
- **Benefits**: Improves circulation and helps resolve discoloration.

4. Apple Cider Vinegar Compress for Healing

- **Ingredients**: 1 tbsp apple cider vinegar, 1 cup warm water, a clean cloth.
- **Method**: Mix vinegar with water, soak the cloth, and apply to the affected area.
- **Benefits**: Improves circulation and promotes healing.

5. Witch Hazel for Bruise Pain

- **Ingredients**: 1 tsp witch hazel.
- **Method**: Dab witch hazel on the bruise using a cotton ball. Repeat 2–3 times daily.
- **Benefits**: Reduces inflammation and alleviates pain.

6. Epsom Salt Soak for Sprains

- **Ingredients**: 1/2 cup Epsom salt, warm water.
- **Method**: Dissolve Epsom salt in warm water and soak the sprained area for 15–20 minutes.
- **Benefits**: Relaxes muscles, reduces swelling, and alleviates pain.

7. Cabbage Compress for Swelling

- **Ingredients**: 2 cabbage leaves.
- **Method**: Slightly crush the cabbage leaves, wrap them around the bruised area, and secure with a bandage.
- **Benefits**: Draws out excess fluid and reduces swelling.

8. Ginger Paste for Sprains

- **Ingredients**: 1-inch fresh ginger (grated), 2 tbsp water.
- **Method**: Grind ginger into a paste and apply to the sprained area. Cover with a cloth for 20 minutes.
- **Benefits**: Reduces inflammation and improves blood flow.

9. Turmeric and Salt Paste for Bruises

- **Ingredients**: 1/2 tsp turmeric powder, 1/4 tsp salt, a few drops of water.
- **Method**: Mix into a paste and apply to the bruise. Leave for 15 minutes before rinsing.
- **Benefits**: Combines anti-inflammatory and pain-relieving properties.

10. Comfrey Ointment for Bruised Tissue

- **Ingredients**: Store-bought comfrey ointment.

- **Method**: Apply a small amount of ointment to the affected area 2–3 times daily.
- **Benefits**: Encourages tissue repair and reduces pain.

11. Raw Potato Compress for Bruises

- **Ingredients**: 1 raw potato (sliced).
- **Method**: Place a slice of raw potato on the bruise and leave for 20 minutes.
- **Benefits**: Draws out heat and reduces discoloration.

12. Cayenne and Coconut Oil Rub for Sprains

- **Ingredients**: 1/4 tsp cayenne powder, 1 tbsp coconut oil.
- **Method**: Mix and gently rub onto the sprain. Avoid broken skin.
- **Benefits**: Increases circulation and reduces pain.

13. Peppermint Essential Oil for Pain Relief

- **Ingredients**: 2 drops peppermint essential oil, 1 tsp olive oil.
- **Method**: Mix and massage onto the bruised or sprained area.
- **Benefits**: Provides a cooling effect and reduces inflammation.

14. Onion Poultice for Bruises

- **Ingredients**: 1 small onion, a clean cloth.
- **Method**: Crush the onion into a pulp, wrap in a cloth, and place on the bruise for 15 minutes.
- **Benefits**: Reduces swelling and improves circulation.

15. Clove Oil for Sprains

- **Ingredients**: 1 drop clove essential oil, 1 tsp carrier oil (e.g., coconut oil).
- **Method**: Mix and gently massage onto the sprain.
- **Benefits**: Reduces pain and promotes relaxation of the affected area.

16. Banana Peel Compress for Bruises

- **Ingredients**: 1 piece of banana peel.
- **Method**: Place the inside of the peel on the bruise and leave for 15 minutes.
- **Benefits**: Soothes and reduces discoloration.

17. Ice and Salt Rub for Immediate Relief

- **Ingredients**: Ice cubes, a pinch of salt, a clean cloth.
- **Method**: Wrap ice cubes in a cloth, sprinkle with salt, and apply to the sprain or bruise.
- **Benefits**: Reduces swelling and relieves pain.

18. Calendula Oil Massage for Bruises

- **Ingredients**: 1 tsp calendula oil.
- **Method**: Massage the oil gently onto the affected area 2–3 times daily.
- **Benefits**: Reduces discoloration and promotes healing.

19. Vinegar and Salt Compress for Sprains

- **Ingredients**: 1 tbsp vinegar, 1 tsp salt, 1 cup warm water.
- **Method**: Mix vinegar and salt in water, soak a cloth, and apply to the sprain.
- **Benefits**: Draws out swelling and relieves pain.

20. Basil Leaves for Bruises

- **Ingredients**: 5 fresh basil leaves.
- **Method**: Crush leaves to extract juice and apply directly to the bruise.
- **Benefits**: Reduces swelling and soothes pain.

21. Mustard Oil Massage for Sprains

- **Ingredients**: 1 tbsp mustard oil.
- **Method**: Warm the oil slightly and massage gently onto the sprain.
- **Benefits**: Improves circulation and reduces stiffness.

22. Black Tea Compress for Bruises

- **Ingredients**: 1 black tea bag, 1 cup hot water.
- **Method**: Steep the tea bag, cool slightly, and apply to the bruise.
- **Benefits**: Reduces swelling and improves circulation.

23. Ice Pack with Chamomile Tea for Sprains

- **Ingredients**: 1 cup brewed chamomile tea, ice cubes.
- **Method**: Mix ice with chamomile tea, soak a cloth, and apply to the sprain.

- **Benefits**: Combines cold therapy with anti-inflammatory benefits.

24. Turmeric and Honey Paste for Bruises

- **Ingredients**: 1/2 tsp turmeric powder, 1 tsp honey.
- **Method**: Mix into a paste and apply to the bruise for 20 minutes.
- **Benefits**: Reduces pain and prevents swelling.

25. Warm Castor Oil for Sprains

- **Ingredients**: 1 tbsp castor oil.
- **Method**: Warm the oil and massage gently onto the sprained area.
- **Benefits**: Relieves stiffness and reduces swelling.

26. Mint Leaf Paste for Bruises

- **Ingredients**: 5 fresh mint leaves.
- **Method**: Crush into a paste and apply to the bruise for 15 minutes.
- **Benefits**: Provides a cooling effect and reduces discoloration.

27. Slippery Elm Powder for Sprains

- **Ingredients**: 1 tsp slippery elm powder, a few drops of water.
- **Method**: Mix into a paste and apply to the sprain. Cover with a cloth.
- **Benefits**: Soothes pain and reduces inflammation.

28. Beetroot Juice for Bruises

- **Ingredients**: 1 tsp fresh beetroot juice.
- **Method**: Dab juice onto the bruise with a cotton ball.
- **Benefits**: Improves blood flow and reduces discoloration.

29. Garlic and Olive Oil Rub for Sprains

- **Ingredients**: 1 clove garlic (crushed), 1 tbsp olive oil.
- **Method**: Mix garlic with olive oil and massage onto the sprain.
- **Benefits**: Relieves pain and prevents swelling.

30. Rosewater and Glycerin Mix for Bruises

- **Ingredients**: 1 tsp rosewater, 1/2 tsp glycerin.
- **Method**: Mix and dab onto the bruise with a cotton ball.
- **Benefits**: Reduces discoloration and soothes the skin.

3.8 Household and Everyday Uses

Natural Cleaning

1. Lemon and Vinegar All-Purpose Cleaner

- **Ingredients**: Peel of 2 lemons, 1 cup white vinegar, 1 cup water.
- **Method**: Soak lemon peels in vinegar for 2 weeks. Strain and dilute with water. Use in a spray bottle for surfaces.
- **Benefits**: Cuts grease, removes stains, and leaves a fresh citrus scent.

2. Baking Soda and Lavender Carpet Freshener

- **Ingredients**: 1 cup baking soda, 10 drops lavender essential oil.
- **Method**: Mix ingredients, sprinkle on carpets, let sit for 15 minutes, and vacuum.
- **Benefits**: Absorbs odors and leaves a calming lavender scent.

3. Rosemary and Lemon Wood Polish

- **Ingredients**: 1/2 cup olive oil, 2 tbsp lemon juice, 5 drops rosemary essential oil.
- **Method**: Mix and apply to wooden furniture with a soft cloth.
- **Benefits**: Cleans, conditions, and shines wood naturally.

4. Tea Tree Bathroom Cleaner

- **Ingredients**: 1 cup water, 1 cup white vinegar, 10 drops tea tree essential oil.
- **Method**: Mix in a spray bottle, spray onto surfaces, and wipe clean.
- **Benefits**: Disinfects and prevents mold and mildew growth.

5. Thyme-Infused Dish Soap

- **Ingredients**: 1/4 cup castile soap, 1 cup water, 5 drops thyme essential oil.
- **Method**: Mix ingredients and use as dish soap.
- **Benefits**: Cuts through grease and kills bacteria.

6. Citrus and Baking Soda Oven Cleaner

- **Ingredients**: 1/2 cup baking soda, juice of 1 lemon, water.
- **Method**: Make a paste, spread on oven surfaces, let sit for 15 minutes, and scrub clean.
- **Benefits**: Removes grease and baked-on stains naturally.

7. Peppermint Glass Cleaner

- **Ingredients**: 1 cup water, 1/4 cup white vinegar, 5 drops peppermint essential oil.
- **Method**: Mix in a spray bottle and use on mirrors and windows.
- **Benefits**: Leaves glass streak-free and smelling fresh.

8. Clove Oil Mold Spray

- **Ingredients**: 1 cup water, 10 drops clove essential oil.
- **Method**: Mix in a spray bottle and apply to moldy areas. Leave for 1 hour, then wipe clean.
- **Benefits**: Kills mold spores and prevents regrowth.

9. Lavender Laundry Freshener

- **Ingredients**: 10 drops lavender essential oil, 1/4 cup baking soda.
- **Method**: Mix and add to the washing machine during the rinse cycle.
- **Benefits**: Naturally softens fabrics and adds a calming scent.

10. Mint and Lemon Sink Scrub

- **Ingredients**: 1/4 cup baking soda, 2 tbsp lemon juice, 5 drops peppermint essential oil.
- **Method**: Make a paste, apply to sinks, scrub, and rinse.
- **Benefits**: Cleans and deodorizes sinks and drains.

11. Epsom Salt Grout Cleaner

- **Ingredients**: 1/4 cup Epsom salt, 1/4 cup baking soda, 1/4 cup warm water.
- **Method**: Mix into a paste, scrub onto grout lines with a toothbrush, and rinse with water.
- **Benefits**: Removes grime and whitens grout naturally.

12. Vinegar and Basil Refrigerator Cleaner

- **Ingredients**: 1/2 cup white vinegar, 1 cup warm water, 5 drops basil essential oil.
- **Method**: Mix ingredients in a spray bottle and wipe refrigerator surfaces.
- **Benefits**: Disinfects and deodorizes while leaving a mild herbal scent.

13. Orange Peel and Cinnamon Garbage Disposal Deodorizer

- **Ingredients**: Peels from 1 orange, 1 tsp ground cinnamon.
- **Method**: Drop orange peels and cinnamon into the disposal, run water, and turn it on.
- **Benefits**: Neutralizes odors and adds a pleasant citrus-spice scent.

14. Pine Needle Floor Cleaner

- **Ingredients**: 1 gallon warm water, 1/2 cup white vinegar, 10 drops pine essential oil.
- **Method**: Mix in a bucket and use to mop floors.
- **Benefits**: Cleans, disinfects, and leaves a fresh, woodsy aroma.

15. Baking Soda Mattress Deodorizer

- **Ingredients**: 1/2 cup baking soda, 5 drops lavender essential oil.
- **Method**: Sprinkle on the mattress, leave for 30 minutes, and vacuum.
- **Benefits**: Neutralizes odors and freshens up mattresses.

16. Lemon and Salt Cutting Board Scrub

- **Ingredients**: Juice of 1 lemon, 1 tbsp salt.
- **Method**: Scrub the cutting board with the mixture, let sit for 5 minutes, and rinse.
- **Benefits**: Disinfects and removes stains and odors.

17. Vinegar and Baking Soda Drain Cleaner

- **Ingredients**: 1/2 cup baking soda, 1 cup vinegar, boiling water.
- **Method**: Pour baking soda into the drain, follow with vinegar, let fizz, and flush with boiling water.
- **Benefits**: Clears clogs and removes drain odors.

18. Peppermint and Vinegar Ant Deterrent

- **Ingredients**: 1 cup white vinegar, 10 drops peppermint essential oil.
- **Method**: Mix in a spray bottle and spray entry points or along ant trails.
- **Benefits**: Repels ants naturally without harmful chemicals.

19. Clove and Cinnamon Toilet Bowl Cleaner

- **Ingredients**: 1/4 cup baking soda, 1/4 cup white vinegar, 5 drops clove essential oil, 5 drops cinnamon essential oil.
- **Method**: Sprinkle baking soda in the bowl, add vinegar and essential oils, and scrub.
- **Benefits**: Disinfects, removes stains, and leaves a warm, spicy scent.

20. Sage and Vinegar Stove Degreaser

- **Ingredients**: 1/2 cup white vinegar, 1 cup water, 5 drops sage essential oil.
- **Method**: Mix in a spray bottle, spray on greasy surfaces, and wipe clean.
- **Benefits**: Cuts through tough grease and disinfects.

21. Thyme and Lemon Microwave Cleaner

- **Ingredients**: 1 cup water, juice of 1 lemon, 5 drops thyme essential oil.
- **Method**: Microwave the mixture for 2 minutes, then wipe down the microwave interior.
- **Benefits**: Loosens grime and leaves a fresh scent.

22. Rosemary Vinegar Stainless Steel Polish

- **Ingredients**: 1/2 cup white vinegar, 10 drops rosemary essential oil, 1 cup water.
- **Method**: Mix in a spray bottle and wipe stainless steel surfaces with a microfiber cloth.
- **Benefits**: Removes smudges and restores shine.

23. DIY Herbal Soap Scum Remover

- **Ingredients**: 1/4 cup castile soap, 1/4 cup baking soda, 5 drops lavender essential oil.
- **Method**: Mix into a paste, apply to soap scum, scrub, and rinse.
- **Benefits**: Cleans bathtubs, tiles, and shower doors.

24. Clove and Lemon Laundry Disinfectant

- **Ingredients**: 10 drops clove essential oil, 10 drops lemon essential oil, 1/4 cup baking soda.
- **Method**: Add the mixture to the washing machine during the rinse cycle.
- **Benefits**: Disinfects and adds a refreshing scent to laundry.

25. Dried Herb Drawer Sachets

- **Ingredients**: 1/2 cup dried lavender, 1/2 cup dried chamomile, fabric pouches.
- **Method**: Fill pouches with dried herbs and place in drawers.

- **Benefits**: Freshens clothes and repels moths naturally.

26. Basil and Mint Window Cleaner

- **Ingredients**: 1/4 cup white vinegar, 1 cup water, 5 drops basil essential oil, 5 drops mint essential oil.
- **Method**: Mix in a spray bottle and use on windows or mirrors.
- **Benefits**: Leaves glass streak-free with a refreshing scent.

27. Grapefruit and Salt Bathtub Scrub

- **Ingredients**: 1/2 grapefruit (sliced), 1/4 cup salt.
- **Method**: Use the grapefruit slice as a scrubber, dipped in salt, to clean the bathtub.
- **Benefits**: Removes grime and leaves a fruity aroma.

28. Citrus Vinegar Fridge Deodorizer

- **Ingredients**: Peels of 2 oranges, 1 cup white vinegar, 1 cup water.
- **Method**: Mix ingredients in a spray bottle, clean fridge shelves, and wipe with a damp cloth.
- **Benefits**: Disinfects and removes fridge odors.

29. Pine and Rosemary Floor Freshener

- **Ingredients**: 1 gallon warm water, 10 drops pine essential oil, 10 drops rosemary essential oil.
- **Method**: Mix and mop floors.
- **Benefits**: Cleans and leaves a fresh, woodsy scent.

30. DIY Citrus Garbage Can Wipe

- **Ingredients**: 1/4 cup white vinegar, juice of 1 lemon, 1 cup water.
- **Method**: Mix and use with a cloth to wipe garbage cans.
- **Benefits**: Removes odors and disinfects naturally.

Air Fresheners and Mists

1. Lavender and Citrus Room Spray

- **Ingredients**: 1 cup distilled water, 10 drops lavender essential oil, 5 drops orange essential oil.

- **Method**: Mix in a spray bottle and mist around the room.
- **Best For**: A calming and refreshing floral-citrus scent.

2. Mint and Rosemary Simmering Pot

- **Ingredients**: 1 sprig rosemary, a handful of mint leaves, 2 cups water.
- **Method**: Simmer ingredients on the stovetop, adding water as needed.
- **Best For**: Neutralizing odors and creating a fresh herbal aroma.

3. Cinnamon and Clove Stovetop Potpourri

- **Ingredients**: 2 cinnamon sticks, 1 tbsp cloves, 1 orange peel, 2 cups water.
- **Method**: Simmer ingredients on the stovetop for a warm, spicy scent.
- **Best For**: Cozy fall or winter ambiance.

4. Basil and Lemon Room Mist

- **Ingredients**: 1 cup distilled water, 10 drops basil essential oil, 5 drops lemon essential oil.
- **Method**: Mix in a spray bottle and mist as needed.
- **Best For**: A fresh, herbal-citrus scent to energize your home.

5. Vanilla and Peppermint Spray

- **Ingredients**: 1 cup water, 1 tsp vanilla extract, 5 drops peppermint essential oil.
- **Method**: Mix in a spray bottle and use to freshen rooms.
- **Best For**: A sweet and minty scent to invigorate the senses.

6. Dried Lavender and Chamomile Sachets

- **Ingredients**: 1/2 cup dried lavender, 1/2 cup dried chamomile, small fabric pouches.
- **Method**: Fill pouches with herbs and place in drawers, closets, or under pillows.
- **Best For**: Gentle floral fragrance to freshen linens and small spaces.

7. Grapefruit and Mint Diffuser Blend

- **Ingredients**: 5 drops grapefruit essential oil, 5 drops peppermint essential oil.
- **Method**: Add to a diffuser with water and run in any room.
- **Best For**: An uplifting and energizing aroma.

8. Rose and Geranium Mist

- **Ingredients**: 1 cup distilled water, 5 drops rose essential oil, 5 drops geranium essential oil.
- **Method**: Mix in a spray bottle and mist lightly.
- **Best For**: A romantic and floral scent for bedrooms or living spaces.

9. Vanilla and Cinnamon Potpourri

- **Ingredients**: 1/4 cup dried orange peels, 1 tbsp cinnamon sticks, 1 tsp vanilla extract.
- **Method**: Combine ingredients in a decorative bowl.
- **Best For**: A warm and inviting scent for kitchens and dining areas.

10. Citrus and Eucalyptus Room Spray

- **Ingredients**: 1 cup distilled water, 10 drops orange essential oil, 5 drops eucalyptus essential oil.
- **Method**: Mix in a spray bottle and use as needed.
- **Best For**: A clean and refreshing scent for bathrooms or kitchens.

11. Dried Herb and Citrus Potpourri

- **Ingredients**: Dried rosemary, thyme, and basil leaves, mixed with lemon zest.
- **Method**: Combine in a bowl or sachet for closets or countertops.
- **Best For**: A fresh herbal aroma that gently fills the air.

12. Pine and Cedarwood Diffuser Blend

- **Ingredients**: 5 drops pine essential oil, 5 drops cedarwood essential oil.
- **Method**: Add to a diffuser with water and run in any room.
- **Best For**: A woodsy, outdoor-inspired scent.

13. Rose and Orange Mist

- **Ingredients**: 1 cup distilled water, 5 drops rose essential oil, 5 drops orange essential oil.
- **Method**: Mix in a spray bottle and mist throughout the home.
- **Best For**: A floral-citrus scent that uplifts and refreshes.

14. Chamomile and Lavender Linen Spray

- **Ingredients**: 1 cup water, 5 drops chamomile essential oil, 5 drops lavender essential oil.
- **Method**: Mix in a spray bottle and use to freshen linens.

- **Best For**: Relaxing bedtime scent for sheets and pillowcases.

15. Lemon Balm Simmer Pot

- **Ingredients**: 1/2 cup fresh lemon balm leaves, 2 cups water.
- **Method**: Simmer on the stovetop for a fresh lemony aroma.
- **Best For**: Naturally freshening the kitchen or living areas.

16. Sage and Lavender Smudge Stick

- **Ingredients**: Fresh sage leaves, lavender sprigs, and twine.
- **Method**: Tie herbs together, let dry, and burn gently to release fragrance.
- **Best For**: Purifying the air and adding a subtle herbal aroma.

17. Orange and Clove Diffuser Blend

- **Ingredients**: 5 drops orange essential oil, 5 drops clove essential oil.
- **Method**: Add to a diffuser with water and run in any room.
- **Best For**: A warm, spicy-citrus scent for holiday or winter months.

18. Peppermint and Rosemary Room Spray

- **Ingredients**: 1 cup distilled water, 5 drops peppermint essential oil, 5 drops rosemary essential oil.
- **Method**: Mix in a spray bottle and mist around the room.
- **Best For**: A sharp, clean scent to energize and refresh.

19. Eucalyptus and Lime Shower Mist

- **Ingredients**: 1 cup distilled water, 10 drops eucalyptus essential oil, 5 drops lime essential oil.
- **Method**: Mix in a spray bottle and spritz in the shower for a spa-like effect.
- **Best For**: A refreshing, invigorating aroma.

20. Cinnamon and Vanilla Stove Simmer

- **Ingredients**: 2 cinnamon sticks, 1 tsp vanilla extract, 2 cups water.
- **Method**: Simmer on the stove for a cozy aroma.
- **Best For**: Adding warmth and comfort to your home.

21. Dried Flower Potpourri

- **Ingredients**: Dried rose petals, lavender buds, chamomile flowers, and orange zest.
- **Method**: Mix and place in a decorative bowl.
- **Best For**: A gentle floral and citrus fragrance.

22. Mint and Lemon Peel Simmer Pot

- **Ingredients**: A handful of mint leaves, peel of 1 lemon, 2 cups water.
- **Method**: Simmer on the stovetop for a refreshing scent.
- **Best For**: Neutralizing kitchen odors.

23. Clove and Pine Diffuser Blend

- **Ingredients**: 5 drops clove essential oil, 5 drops pine essential oil.
- **Method**: Add to a diffuser with water and run in living spaces.
- **Best For**: A cozy, woodsy scent for colder seasons.

24. Vanilla and Lavender Drawer Sachets

- **Ingredients**: Dried lavender, a few drops vanilla essential oil, small fabric pouches.
- **Method**: Mix and place sachets in drawers or closets.
- **Best For**: Subtly freshening clothes and linens.

25. Grapefruit and Basil Spray

- **Ingredients**: 1 cup distilled water, 5 drops grapefruit essential oil, 5 drops basil essential oil.
- **Method**: Mix in a spray bottle and mist as needed.
- **Best For**: Uplifting and freshening living spaces.

26. Mint and Pine Floor Cleaner Aroma

- **Ingredients**: 1 gallon warm water, 10 drops mint essential oil, 5 drops pine essential oil.
- **Method**: Mix in a bucket and use to mop floors.
- **Best For**: Cleaning floors while releasing a fresh scent.

27. Orange and Thyme Simmer Pot

- **Ingredients**: Orange slices, 2 sprigs thyme, 2 cups water.
- **Method**: Simmer on the stovetop to fill the room with fragrance.
- **Best For**: A citrus-herbal aroma for kitchens and dining areas.

28. Lemon and Basil Spray

- **Ingredients**: 1 cup distilled water, 10 drops lemon essential oil, 5 drops basil essential oil.
- **Method**: Mix in a spray bottle and mist around the home.
- **Best For**: Freshening up bathrooms or kitchens.

29. Chamomile and Eucalyptus Diffuser Blend

- **Ingredients**: 5 drops chamomile essential oil, 5 drops eucalyptus essential oil.
- **Method**: Add to a diffuser with water and run.
- **Best For**: Creating a calming and refreshing atmosphere.

30. Vanilla Bean and Clove Simmer Pot

- **Ingredients**: 1 vanilla bean (split), 1 tbsp cloves, 2 cups water.
- **Method**: Simmer on the stovetop for a sweet, spicy aroma.
- **Best For**: A cozy and comforting scent.

Insect and Pest Control

1. Citronella and Eucalyptus Bug Spray

- **Ingredients**: 1 cup water, 10 drops citronella essential oil, 5 drops eucalyptus essential oil.
- **Method**: Mix in a spray bottle and apply to exposed skin or outdoor areas.
- **Best For**: Repelling mosquitoes and outdoor bugs.

2. Basil Leaf Mosquito Repellent

- **Ingredients**: A handful of fresh basil leaves, 1 cup water.
- **Method**: Simmer basil leaves in water for 10 minutes, cool, and strain. Spray around mosquito-prone areas.
- **Best For**: Keeping mosquitoes away naturally.

3. Peppermint and Vinegar Ant Deterrent

- **Ingredients**: 1 cup white vinegar, 10 drops peppermint essential oil.
- **Method**: Mix in a spray bottle and mist along ant trails and entry points.
- **Best For**: Repelling ants from kitchens and pantries.

4. Clove and Lemon Ant Repellent

- **Ingredients**: 10 whole cloves, 1 lemon (sliced).
- **Method**: Press cloves into lemon slices and place them in ant-prone areas.
- **Best For**: Naturally deterring ants with a strong scent.

5. Lavender and Rosemary Fly Spray

- **Ingredients**: 1 cup water, 10 drops lavender essential oil, 5 drops rosemary essential oil.
- **Method**: Mix in a spray bottle and mist in fly-prone areas.
- **Best For**: Keeping flies out of kitchens and dining rooms.

6. Neem Oil Spray for Garden Pests

- **Ingredients**: 1 tbsp neem oil, 1 tsp dish soap, 1 liter water.
- **Method**: Mix and spray on plants to deter aphids, whiteflies, and other pests.
- **Best For**: Protecting indoor and outdoor plants.

7. Garlic and Chili Spray for Outdoor Insects

- **Ingredients**: 2 garlic cloves, 1 tsp chili powder, 1 liter water.
- **Method**: Blend garlic and chili with water, strain, and spray on plants.
- **Best For**: Repelling beetles, caterpillars, and other garden pests.

8. Dried Bay Leaves for Pantry Moths

- **Ingredients**: A few dried bay leaves.
- **Method**: Place bay leaves on pantry shelves or inside food containers.
- **Best For**: Keeping pantry moths and other bugs away from food.

9. Lemon Balm Mosquito Repellent

- **Ingredients**: Fresh lemon balm leaves.
- **Method**: Crush the leaves to release their oils and rub onto skin or place near windows.
- **Best For**: Repelling mosquitoes naturally.

10. Cedarwood Chips for Moths

- **Ingredients**: Cedarwood chips or balls.

- **Method**: Place cedarwood in closets or drawers.
- **Best For**: Repelling moths and keeping clothes fresh.

11. Vinegar and Peppermint Spider Spray

- **Ingredients**: 1 cup vinegar, 10 drops peppermint essential oil.
- **Method**: Mix in a spray bottle and apply to spider-prone corners and cracks.
- **Best For**: Preventing spider webs indoors.

12. Orange Peel Fly Deterrent

- **Ingredients**: Fresh orange peels.
- **Method**: Place peels near windows or kitchen counters to repel flies.
- **Best For**: Keeping flies out of the kitchen.

13. Coffee Grounds for Garden Pests

- **Ingredients**: Used coffee grounds.
- **Method**: Sprinkle coffee grounds around plants.
- **Best For**: Deterring snails, slugs, and ants from gardens.

14. Rosemary Smoke for Mosquitoes

- **Ingredients**: Fresh rosemary sprigs.
- **Method**: Toss rosemary on a grill or firepit to create mosquito-repelling smoke.
- **Best For**: Outdoor gatherings in mosquito-prone areas.

15. Lavender Sachets for Drawers

- **Ingredients**: Dried lavender flowers, small fabric pouches.
- **Method**: Fill pouches and place in drawers or closets.
- **Best For**: Repelling moths and freshening clothes.

16. Mint and Vinegar Ant Spray

- **Ingredients**: 1 cup vinegar, 10 drops mint essential oil.
- **Method**: Mix in a spray bottle and spray along ant trails.
- **Best For**: Creating a natural barrier to repel ants.

17. Lemon Eucalyptus Mosquito Lotion

- **Ingredients**: 10 drops lemon eucalyptus essential oil, 1 tbsp coconut oil.
- **Method**: Mix and apply to exposed skin.
- **Best For**: Preventing mosquito bites.

18. Thyme and Clove Garden Spray

- **Ingredients**: 1 cup water, 5 drops thyme essential oil, 5 drops clove essential oil.
- **Method**: Mix and spray on garden plants to repel pests.
- **Best For**: Protecting vegetable gardens from insects.

19. Basil Planter for Mosquito Control

- **Ingredients**: Potted basil plant.
- **Method**: Place the plant near seating areas outdoors.
- **Best For**: Keeping mosquitoes at bay naturally.

20. Chamomile Spray for Fleas

- **Ingredients**: 1 cup brewed chamomile tea, spray bottle.
- **Method**: Cool the tea, pour into a spray bottle, and spray on pet bedding or carpets.
- **Best For**: Repelling fleas and freshening pet areas.

21. Clove and Cinnamon Fly Spray

- **Ingredients**: 1 cup water, 5 drops clove essential oil, 5 drops cinnamon essential oil.
- **Method**: Mix in a spray bottle and mist in fly-prone areas.
- **Best For**: Keeping flies out of living spaces.

22. Mint and Lemon Plant Watering Spray

- **Ingredients**: 1 liter water, 5 drops mint essential oil, 5 drops lemon essential oil.
- **Method**: Mix and spray on plants to deter pests.
- **Best For**: Repelling aphids and keeping plants healthy.

23. Vanilla and Citrus Mosquito Spray

- **Ingredients**: 1 cup water, 1 tsp vanilla extract, 10 drops orange essential oil.
- **Method**: Mix in a spray bottle and mist around outdoor areas.

- **Best For**: Creating a mosquito-free outdoor space.

24. Eucalyptus and Lavender Dog Collar

- **Ingredients**: 2 drops eucalyptus essential oil, 2 drops lavender essential oil, a cotton dog collar.
- **Method**: Add oils to the collar and let dry before putting it on your pet.
- **Best For**: Repelling fleas and ticks.

25. Garlic and Mint Garden Spray

- **Ingredients**: 1 garlic clove, a handful of mint leaves, 1 liter water.
- **Method**: Blend ingredients, strain, and spray on garden plants.
- **Best For**: Repelling garden pests naturally.

26. Tea Tree Oil Flea Spray

- **Ingredients**: 1 cup water, 5 drops tea tree essential oil.
- **Method**: Mix and spray on pet bedding or carpets.
- **Best For**: Repelling fleas and freshening spaces.

27. Lemon Vinegar Wasp Deterrent

- **Ingredients**: 1/2 cup vinegar, juice of 1 lemon, 1 cup water.
- **Method**: Mix and spray near wasp nests (from a safe distance).
- **Best For**: Keeping wasps away from patios and outdoor areas.

28. Mint and Rosemary Fly Strips

- **Ingredients**: 1 cup water, 5 drops mint essential oil, 5 drops rosemary essential oil, strips of cloth.
- **Method**: Soak cloth strips in the mixture and hang them in fly-prone areas.
- **Best For**: Reducing fly presence indoors and outdoors.

29. Onion Water Spider Spray

- **Ingredients**: 1 onion (blended), 1 cup water.
- **Method**: Blend onion with water, strain, and spray in spider-prone areas.
- **Best For**: Preventing spiders in corners and crevices.

30. Bay Leaf and Citrus Pantry Spray

- **Ingredients**: 1 cup water, 10 drops orange essential oil, a few crushed bay leaves.
- **Method**: Mix and spray shelves and pantry areas.
- **Best For**: Keeping pantry bugs and moths away naturally.

3.9 Seasonal Wellness and Remedies

Spring Renewal

1. Nettle Leaf Compress for Allergy Relief

- **Ingredients**: Fresh or dried nettle leaves, hot water, a clean cloth.
- **Method**: Soak nettle leaves in hot water, strain, and soak the cloth in the liquid. Apply to itchy or irritated areas.
- **Benefits**: Reduces itching and inflammation caused by seasonal allergies.

2. Eucalyptus Steam Bath for Sinus Congestion

- **Ingredients**: A few fresh eucalyptus leaves or 5 drops eucalyptus essential oil, hot water.
- **Method**: Add eucalyptus to hot bathwater and soak while inhaling the steam.
- **Benefits**: Opens nasal passages and clears sinuses.

3. Dry Brushing for Detoxification

- **Ingredients**: A natural bristle brush.
- **Method**: Brush the skin gently in upward strokes before showering, starting at the feet and moving toward the heart.
- **Benefits**: Stimulates lymphatic drainage and exfoliates the skin.

4. Herbal Eye Pillow for Allergy Relief

- **Ingredients**: Dried lavender, chamomile, and a small fabric pouch.
- **Method**: Fill the pouch with dried herbs and place over your eyes while lying down.
- **Benefits**: Soothes irritated eyes and reduces puffiness caused by allergies.

5. Spring Herb Infused Oil for Skin Health

- **Ingredients**: Fresh dandelion flowers, olive oil, glass jar.
- **Method**: Fill the jar with dandelion flowers, cover with olive oil, and let infuse in sunlight for 2 weeks. Strain and apply to skin.
- **Benefits**: Moisturizes and soothes dry or irritated skin.

6. Detoxifying Foot Soak with Epsom Salt

- **Ingredients**: 1/2 cup Epsom salt, juice of 1 lemon, warm water.
- **Method**: Soak feet in the mixture for 20 minutes.
- **Benefits**: Draws out toxins and relieves tired feet.

7. Turmeric and Aloe Face Mask for Skin Renewal

- **Ingredients**: 1 tsp turmeric powder, 2 tbsp aloe vera gel.
- **Method**: Mix ingredients, apply to the face, and leave on for 15 minutes. Rinse with warm water.
- **Benefits**: Brightens skin and reduces inflammation.

8. Basil and Mint Pollen Defense Balm

- **Ingredients**: 2 tbsp coconut oil, 5 drops basil essential oil, 5 drops mint essential oil.
- **Method**: Mix and apply under the nose to block pollen.
- **Benefits**: Eases allergy symptoms and protects against pollen exposure.

9. Spring Detox Bath with Dried Herbs

- **Ingredients**: 1/2 cup dried chamomile, 1/2 cup dried rosemary, 1/2 cup dried lavender, cheesecloth.
- **Method**: Place herbs in cheesecloth, tie securely, and toss into warm bathwater. Soak for 20 minutes.
- **Benefits**: Promotes relaxation and detoxifies the skin.

10. Fennel and Peppermint Digestive Compress

- **Ingredients**: 1 tsp fennel seeds, 1 tsp dried peppermint, hot water, clean cloth.
- **Method**: Brew fennel and peppermint in hot water, soak the cloth, and apply to the abdomen.
- **Benefits**: Relieves bloating and aids digestion.

11. Lavender Pillow Sachets for Better Sleep

- **Ingredients**: Dried lavender, small fabric pouches.
- **Method**: Fill pouches with lavender and place them under your pillow.
- **Benefits**: Encourages restful sleep and reduces springtime restlessness.

12. Peppermint Essential Oil Massage for Fatigue

- **Ingredients**: 1 tbsp carrier oil (coconut or almond oil), 2 drops peppermint essential oil.
- **Method**: Mix oils and massage onto temples and the back of the neck.
- **Benefits**: Boosts energy and reduces fatigue.

13. Chamomile Eye Compress for Irritation

- **Ingredients**: 2 chamomile tea bags, warm water.
- **Method**: Soak tea bags in warm water, cool slightly, and place over closed eyes for 10 minutes.
- **Benefits**: Reduces redness and itching caused by spring allergens.

14. Parsley Poultice for Puffy Eyes

- **Ingredients**: Fresh parsley, a clean cloth.
- **Method**: Crush parsley into a paste, wrap in the cloth, and place over eyes for 10 minutes.
- **Benefits**: Reduces puffiness and soothes tired eyes.

15. Herbal Vinegar Hair Rinse for Shine

- **Ingredients**: 1 cup apple cider vinegar, 1/2 cup fresh rosemary or mint leaves.
- **Method**: Infuse herbs in vinegar for 1 week, strain, and dilute with water. Use as a final rinse after shampooing.
- **Benefits**: Restores scalp health and adds shine to hair.

16. Lemon Balm Hand Scrub for Dry Skin

- **Ingredients**: 1/4 cup sugar, 2 tbsp olive oil, 5 drops lemon balm essential oil.
- **Method**: Mix ingredients and massage onto hands before rinsing.
- **Benefits**: Exfoliates and hydrates hands after winter dryness.

17. Mustard Foot Paste for Circulation

- **Ingredients**: 1 tsp mustard powder, warm water.
- **Method**: Mix into a paste and apply to the soles of the feet for 10 minutes. Rinse thoroughly.
- **Benefits**: Stimulates circulation and reduces sluggishness.

18. Calendula Salve for Irritated Skin

- **Ingredients**: 1/4 cup calendula-infused oil, 1 tbsp beeswax.
- **Method**: Melt beeswax, mix with calendula oil, and store in a jar. Apply to irritated skin.

- **Benefits**: Soothes skin irritation caused by spring allergens.

19. Aloe and Mint Cooling Gel for Itchy Skin

- **Ingredients**: 2 tbsp aloe vera gel, 5 drops peppermint essential oil.
- **Method**: Mix and apply to itchy or irritated areas.
- **Benefits**: Soothes skin and provides a cooling effect.

20. Spring Green Clay Mask for Detox

- **Ingredients**: 1 tbsp green clay, 1 tbsp water, 2 drops rosemary essential oil.
- **Method**: Mix into a paste, apply to the face, and leave for 10 minutes before rinsing.
- **Benefits**: Draws out impurities and refreshes skin.

21. Herbal Body Oil Massage for Detox

- **Ingredients**: 1/2 cup sesame oil, 10 drops lemongrass essential oil.
- **Method**: Warm the oil slightly and massage onto the body before showering.
- **Benefits**: Improves lymphatic flow and detoxifies the skin.

22. Mint and Eucalyptus Diffuser Blend for Refreshing the Home

- **Ingredients**: 5 drops mint essential oil, 5 drops eucalyptus essential oil, a diffuser.
- **Method**: Add oils to a diffuser and run in any room.
- **Benefits**: Clears the air and boosts energy.

23. Elderflower Infused Vinegar for Allergies

- **Ingredients**: Fresh elderflowers, apple cider vinegar.
- **Method**: Infuse elderflowers in vinegar for 2 weeks, strain, and store. Dilute with water for cleaning or skincare.
- **Benefits**: Soothes skin and supports seasonal allergy relief.

24. Ginger Compress for Muscle Tension Relief

- **Ingredients**: 2 tbsp grated ginger, 1 quart hot water, a clean cloth.
- **Method**: Soak the cloth in ginger-infused hot water, wring out excess liquid, and apply to tense or sore muscles for 15 minutes.
- **Benefits**: Improves circulation, relieves muscle tension, and reduces inflammation.

25. Wildflower and Herb Sachets for Stress Relief

- **Ingredients**: A mix of dried lavender, chamomile, and rose petals, small fabric pouches.
- **Method**: Fill the pouches with the herbs and keep them in your workspace, living room, or car.
- **Benefits**: Provides a calming scent to reduce stress and refresh your environment.

Summer Cooling and Protection

1. Cucumber and Aloe Cooling Face Mask

- **Ingredients**: 2 tbsp aloe vera gel, 2 tbsp grated cucumber.
- **Method**: Mix aloe and cucumber into a smooth paste, apply to your face, and leave for 15 minutes. Rinse with cool water.
- **Benefits**: Soothes sunburn, reduces redness, and cools overheated skin.

2. Peppermint and Lemon Foot Soak for Heat Relief

- **Ingredients**: 5 drops peppermint essential oil, juice of 1 lemon, warm water.
- **Method**: Add ingredients to a basin of water and soak feet for 15 minutes.
- **Benefits**: Cools tired feet and reduces swelling after a hot day.

3. Coconut Oil and Mint Cooling Hair Mask

- **Ingredients**: 2 tbsp coconut oil, 5 drops peppermint essential oil.
- **Method**: Mix and apply to your scalp and hair. Leave for 30 minutes and rinse thoroughly.
- **Benefits**: Hydrates the scalp, cools the head, and protects hair from heat damage.

4. Rosewater Facial Mist for Instant Cooling

- **Ingredients**: 1/2 cup rosewater, 5 drops lavender essential oil, spray bottle.
- **Method**: Mix in a spray bottle and spritz on your face as needed.
- **Benefits**: Refreshes skin, soothes irritation, and hydrates on hot days.

5. Hibiscus and Aloe After-Sun Gel

- **Ingredients**: 2 tbsp aloe vera gel, 1 tbsp hibiscus powder.
- **Method**: Mix into a gel and apply to sun-exposed skin. Leave on for 20 minutes and rinse.
- **Benefits**: Cools and repairs sun-damaged skin while reducing inflammation.

6. Mint and Lime Infused Water for Hydration

- **Ingredients**: 5 mint leaves, 3 lime slices, 1 liter water.
- **Method**: Add mint and lime to water, chill, and sip throughout the day.
- **Benefits**: Keeps the body hydrated and cool.

7. Calendula and Chamomile Soothing Compress

- **Ingredients**: 1 tsp dried calendula flowers, 1 tsp dried chamomile, hot water, a clean cloth.
- **Method**: Steep flowers in hot water for 10 minutes, soak the cloth, and apply to sunburned areas.
- **Benefits**: Reduces redness and soothes skin irritation.

8. Basil and Sandalwood Cooling Body Powder

- **Ingredients**: 1/2 cup cornstarch, 1 tsp dried basil powder, 1 tsp sandalwood powder.
- **Method**: Mix ingredients and dust onto the body after a shower.
- **Benefits**: Absorbs sweat and leaves the skin feeling cool and refreshed.

9. Aloe Vera Ice Cubes for Sunburn Relief

- **Ingredients**: Fresh aloe vera gel.
- **Method**: Pour aloe vera gel into an ice cube tray and freeze. Rub cubes on sunburned skin as needed.
- **Benefits**: Provides instant cooling and soothes irritated skin.

10. Lemon Balm and Peppermint Face Compress

- **Ingredients**: A handful of fresh lemon balm and peppermint leaves, hot water, a clean cloth.
- **Method**: Steep herbs in hot water, cool slightly, soak the cloth, and apply to the face.
- **Benefits**: Refreshes and cools overheated skin.

11. Herbal Deodorant Spray

- **Ingredients**: 1/2 cup witch hazel, 10 drops tea tree oil, 10 drops lavender oil, spray bottle.
- **Method**: Mix in a spray bottle and use underarms as needed.
- **Benefits**: Keeps you fresh while naturally combating odor.

12. Cucumber and Mint Eye Pads

- **Ingredients**: 2 slices of cucumber, 2 fresh mint leaves.
- **Method**: Place mint leaves on the cucumber slices and place over closed eyes for 10 minutes.
- **Benefits**: Reduces puffiness and refreshes tired eyes.

13. Green Tea Body Splash for Heat Rash

- **Ingredients**: 1 cup brewed green tea (cooled).
- **Method**: Pour cooled tea over a clean cloth and dab onto heat rash or irritated areas.
- **Benefits**: Reduces itching and inflammation.

14. Coconut and Aloe Body Lotion

- **Ingredients**: 2 tbsp coconut oil, 1 tbsp aloe vera gel.
- **Method**: Mix and apply to skin after sun exposure.
- **Benefits**: Hydrates and repairs skin.

15. Chamomile Ice Pack for Heat Exhaustion

- **Ingredients**: 2 chamomile tea bags, water, an ice cube tray.
- **Method**: Brew tea, pour into an ice cube tray, and freeze. Wrap cubes in a cloth and apply to the forehead or neck.
- **Benefits**: Reduces body temperature and soothes heat exhaustion symptoms.

16. Neem and Turmeric Body Wash

- **Ingredients**: 1 tsp neem powder, 1 tsp turmeric powder, 1/4 cup water.
- **Method**: Mix into a paste, use as a body wash, and rinse thoroughly.
- **Benefits**: Cools the skin and protects against summer rashes.

17. Peppermint Foot Balm for Cooling

- **Ingredients**: 2 tbsp coconut oil, 5 drops peppermint essential oil, 1 tsp beeswax.
- **Method**: Melt beeswax, mix with coconut oil and peppermint oil, and apply to feet.
- **Benefits**: Cools and soothes tired, overheated feet.

18. Rose and Cucumber Face Toner

- **Ingredients**: 1/4 cup rosewater, 1/4 cup cucumber juice.
- **Method**: Mix and store in a spray bottle. Use as a toner after washing your face.

- **Benefits**: Refreshes and hydrates the skin.

19. Oatmeal Bath for Heat Rash

- **Ingredients**: 1/2 cup oatmeal, cheesecloth.
- **Method**: Wrap oatmeal in cheesecloth, place in warm bathwater, and soak for 20 minutes.
- **Benefits**: Soothes and cools heat rashes.

20. Lemon and Rosemary Scalp Spray

- **Ingredients**: 1 cup water, juice of 1 lemon, 5 drops rosemary essential oil.
- **Method**: Mix and spritz onto the scalp for instant cooling.
- **Benefits**: Refreshes the scalp and prevents itchiness caused by sweat.

21. Aloe and Mint Cooling Gel for Scalp

- **Ingredients**: 2 tbsp aloe vera gel, 5 drops mint essential oil.
- **Method**: Apply to the scalp, leave for 15 minutes, and rinse.
- **Benefits**: Cools and soothes the scalp during hot weather.

22. Herbal Cooling Sachets for Bedding

- **Ingredients**: Dried lavender, chamomile, and mint leaves, small fabric pouches.
- **Method**: Fill pouches and place under pillows or on beds.
- **Benefits**: Keeps bedding smelling fresh and cool.

23. Sandalwood Paste for Prickly Heat

- **Ingredients**: 2 tbsp sandalwood powder, a few drops of rosewater.
- **Method**: Mix into a paste, apply to affected areas, and leave for 20 minutes. Rinse with cool water.
- **Benefits**: Relieves prickly heat and soothes irritated skin.

24. Yogurt and Honey After-Sun Mask

- **Ingredients**: 2 tbsp plain yogurt, 1 tsp honey.
- **Method**: Mix and apply to sun-exposed areas for 15 minutes, then rinse.
- **Benefits**: Cools and repairs sunburned skin.

25. Basil and Peppermint Cooling Balm

- **Ingredients**: 1 tbsp coconut oil, 5 drops basil essential oil, 5 drops peppermint essential oil.
- **Method**: Mix and apply to pulse points like the wrists and neck.
- **Benefits**: Provides a cooling sensation and reduces heat exhaustion.

Autumn Immunity and Transition

1. Elderberry Syrup for Immune Support

- **Ingredients**: 1 cup fresh elderberries, 2 cups water, 1/4 cup honey.
- **Method**: Simmer elderberries in water for 30 minutes, strain, cool, and mix with honey. Take 1 tsp daily.
- **Benefits**: Strengthens the immune system and helps prevent colds and flu.

2. Echinacea Tincture for Early Cold Symptoms

- **Ingredients**: 1 cup dried echinacea, 2 cups alcohol (vodka).
- **Method**: Steep echinacea in alcohol for 4–6 weeks, strain, and store in a dark bottle. Take 10 drops at the first sign of a cold.
- **Benefits**: Boosts immune function and fights infections.

3. Turmeric and Ginger Immune Tea

- **Ingredients**: 1 tsp grated turmeric, 1 tsp grated ginger, 1 cup hot water.
- **Method**: Steep turmeric and ginger in hot water for 10 minutes, strain, and drink.
- **Benefits**: Reduces inflammation and strengthens immunity.

4. Garlic and Honey Remedy for Colds

- **Ingredients**: 3 garlic cloves (minced), 1/4 cup raw honey.
- **Method**: Mix garlic with honey and store in a jar. Take 1 tsp daily.
- **Benefits**: Natural antimicrobial that combats cold symptoms and infections.

5. Lemon and Thyme Steam for Congestion

- **Ingredients**: 1 tbsp fresh thyme, juice of 1 lemon, hot water.
- **Method**: Add thyme and lemon juice to hot water, cover your head with a towel, and inhale the steam for 10 minutes.
- **Benefits**: Clears sinuses and eases respiratory discomfort.

6. Rosehip Infusion for Vitamin C

- **Ingredients**: 1 tbsp dried rosehips, 1 cup boiling water.
- **Method**: Steep rosehips in boiling water for 10 minutes, strain, and drink.
- **Benefits**: Provides a high dose of vitamin C for immune support.

7. Fire Cider for Cold Prevention

- **Ingredients**: 1/2 cup grated horseradish, 1/2 cup grated ginger, 1/4 cup garlic (minced), 1/4 cup onion (minced), 2 cups apple cider vinegar.
- **Method**: Combine all ingredients in a jar, seal, and let steep for 4 weeks. Strain and take 1 tbsp daily.
- **Benefits**: Stimulates circulation, clears sinuses, and boosts immunity.

8. Elderflower Tea for Respiratory Health

- **Ingredients**: 1 tsp dried elderflowers, 1 cup boiling water.
- **Method**: Steep elderflowers in boiling water for 10 minutes, strain, and drink.
- **Benefits**: Relieves congestion and soothes seasonal allergies.

9. Apple Cider Vinegar Tonic for Immunity

- **Ingredients**: 1 tbsp apple cider vinegar, 1 tsp honey, 1 cup warm water.
- **Method**: Mix ingredients and drink daily.
- **Benefits**: Balances pH levels and supports immune health.

10. Ginger Compress for Chest Congestion

- **Ingredients**: 1 tbsp grated ginger, hot water, a clean cloth.
- **Method**: Soak the cloth in ginger-infused hot water, wring out, and place on the chest for 10 minutes.
- **Benefits**: Loosens mucus and eases respiratory discomfort.

11. Cinnamon and Clove Tea for Warming

- **Ingredients**: 1 cinnamon stick, 3 cloves, 1 cup boiling water.
- **Method**: Simmer spices in boiling water for 5 minutes, strain, and drink.
- **Benefits**: Warms the body and boosts circulation.

12. Holy Basil (Tulsi) Tea for Stress Relief

- **Ingredients**: 1 tsp dried holy basil, 1 cup boiling water.
- **Method**: Steep tulsi in boiling water for 10 minutes, strain, and drink.
- **Benefits**: Reduces stress and supports the immune system.

13. Herbal Foot Soak for Detoxification

- **Ingredients**: 1/4 cup Epsom salt, 5 drops eucalyptus oil, warm water.
- **Method**: Soak feet for 20 minutes.
- **Benefits**: Draws out toxins and relieves fatigue.

14. Calendula Salve for Dry Skin

- **Ingredients**: 1/4 cup calendula-infused oil, 1 tbsp beeswax.
- **Method**: Melt beeswax, mix with calendula oil, and store in a jar. Apply to dry skin.
- **Benefits**: Heals and soothes dry, cracked skin during autumn.

15. Elderberry and Cinnamon Lozenges

- **Ingredients**: 1/4 cup elderberry syrup, 1/4 tsp cinnamon powder, 1/4 cup powdered sugar.
- **Method**: Mix ingredients, form into small balls, and let dry.
- **Benefits**: Soothes sore throats and boosts immunity.

16. Mullein Leaf Tea for Cough Relief

- **Ingredients**: 1 tsp dried mullein leaves, 1 cup boiling water.
- **Method**: Steep mullein in boiling water for 10 minutes, strain, and drink.
- **Benefits**: Eases coughs and supports lung health.

17. Oregano Oil Drops for Cold Symptoms

- **Ingredients**: 1 drop oregano essential oil, 1 tbsp olive oil.
- **Method**: Mix and take under the tongue or apply to the soles of the feet.
- **Benefits**: Antimicrobial properties to fight infections.

18. Ginger and Honey Cough Syrup

- **Ingredients**: 1/2 cup grated ginger, 1/4 cup honey, 1 cup water.

- **Method**: Simmer ginger in water for 10 minutes, strain, and mix with honey. Take 1 tsp as needed.
- **Benefits**: Relieves cough and soothes the throat.

19. Apple and Cinnamon Infused Water

- **Ingredients**: 1 sliced apple, 1 cinnamon stick, 1 liter water.
- **Method**: Add ingredients to water, let sit for 1 hour, and drink throughout the day.
- **Benefits**: Hydrates and boosts metabolism.

20. Mustard Plaster for Chest Warmth

- **Ingredients**: 1 tbsp mustard powder, 2 tbsp flour, warm water, a cloth.
- **Method**: Mix into a paste, spread on a cloth, and apply to the chest for 15 minutes.
- **Benefits**: Stimulates circulation and relieves chest congestion.

21. Sage and Thyme Gargle for Sore Throats

- **Ingredients**: 1 tsp dried sage, 1 tsp dried thyme, 1 cup hot water.
- **Method**: Steep herbs in hot water, strain, and gargle 3 times daily.
- **Benefits**: Soothes sore throats and kills bacteria.

22. Lemon and Peppermint Steam Inhalation

- **Ingredients**: 5 drops peppermint essential oil, juice of 1 lemon, hot water.
- **Method**: Add ingredients to a bowl of hot water, cover your head with a towel, and inhale deeply.
- **Benefits**: Clears sinuses and supports respiratory health.

23. Ashwagandha Tea for Strengthening Immunity

- **Ingredients**: 1 tsp ashwagandha powder, 1 cup hot milk or water.
- **Method**: Mix and drink once daily.
- **Benefits**: Builds strength and resilience during seasonal transitions.

24. Lemon Balm Infusion for Restful Sleep

- **Ingredients**: 1 tsp dried lemon balm, 1 cup boiling water.
- **Method**: Steep lemon balm in boiling water for 10 minutes, strain, and drink before bed.
- **Benefits**: Calms the mind and helps with sleep during seasonal changes.

25. Spiced Golden Milk for Warming and Immune Boosting

- **Ingredients**: 1 cup warm milk (or plant-based milk), 1/4 tsp turmeric, 1/4 tsp cinnamon, 1 tsp honey.
- **Method**: Mix all ingredients and drink warm.
- **Benefits**: Supports immunity and provides warmth and comfort.

Winter Warmth and Resilience

1. Ginger and Cinnamon Warming Tea

- **Ingredients**: 1-inch ginger root, 1 cinnamon stick, 1 cup water, honey (optional).
- **Method**: Simmer ginger and cinnamon in water for 10 minutes, strain, and drink warm.
- **Benefits**: Improves circulation, warms the body, and strengthens immunity.

2. Clove and Orange Essential Oil Diffuser Blend

- **Ingredients**: 5 drops clove essential oil, 5 drops orange essential oil, water for diffuser.
- **Method**: Add oils and water to a diffuser and run in your living space.
- **Benefits**: Creates a warm, comforting environment and promotes relaxation.

3. Mustard Foot Soak for Warmth

- **Ingredients**: 1 tbsp mustard powder, warm water, basin.
- **Method**: Mix mustard powder into warm water and soak your feet for 15 minutes.
- **Benefits**: Stimulates circulation and warms the body quickly.

4. Spiced Golden Milk for Immune Support

- **Ingredients**: 1 cup warm milk (or plant-based milk), 1/2 tsp turmeric, 1/4 tsp cinnamon, 1 tsp honey.
- **Method**: Mix all ingredients and drink warm before bed.
- **Benefits**: Combats inflammation and supports the immune system.

5. Eucalyptus Steam for Congestion Relief

- **Ingredients**: 5 drops eucalyptus essential oil, hot water.
- **Method**: Add eucalyptus oil to a bowl of hot water, cover your head with a towel, and inhale the steam for 10 minutes.

- **Benefits**: Clears nasal passages and soothes winter respiratory issues.

6. Garlic and Honey Immune Tonic

- **Ingredients**: 3 minced garlic cloves, 1/4 cup raw honey.
- **Method**: Mix garlic and honey in a jar, let sit for a day, and take 1 tsp daily.
- **Benefits**: Boosts immunity and fights colds.

7. Warming Body Oil with Ginger and Black Pepper

- **Ingredients**: 1/4 cup carrier oil (e.g., almond or coconut oil), 3 drops ginger essential oil, 3 drops black pepper essential oil.
- **Method**: Mix oils and massage onto the body after a shower.
- **Benefits**: Improves circulation and keeps the body warm.

8. Rosemary and Lavender Bath Soak

- **Ingredients**: 1/2 cup Epsom salt, 5 drops rosemary essential oil, 5 drops lavender essential oil.
- **Method**: Add to warm bathwater and soak for 20 minutes.
- **Benefits**: Relaxes muscles, eases winter aches, and improves circulation.

9. Fire Cider for Winter Immunity

- **Ingredients**: 1/4 cup grated ginger, 1/4 cup grated horseradish, 1/4 cup chopped garlic, 2 cups apple cider vinegar.
- **Method**: Combine ingredients in a jar, steep for 4 weeks, strain, and take 1 tbsp daily.
- **Benefits**: Boosts immunity and warms the body.

10. Peppermint and Chamomile Sleep Tea

- **Ingredients**: 1 tsp dried peppermint, 1 tsp dried chamomile, 1 cup boiling water.
- **Method**: Steep herbs in boiling water for 10 minutes, strain, and drink before bed.
- **Benefits**: Promotes restful sleep and reduces winter stress.

11. Warming Soup with Garlic and Turmeric

- **Ingredients**: 2 garlic cloves (minced), 1/2 tsp turmeric, vegetable broth, vegetables of choice.
- **Method**: Simmer garlic and turmeric in broth with vegetables, and enjoy warm.
- **Benefits**: Supports digestion and boosts immunity.

12. Clove and Cinnamon Chest Rub

- **Ingredients**: 1/4 cup coconut oil, 5 drops clove essential oil, 5 drops cinnamon essential oil.
- **Method**: Mix oils and massage onto the chest for warmth and congestion relief.
- **Benefits**: Warms the body and reduces chest tightness.

13. Elderberry and Ginger Syrup for Cold Prevention

- **Ingredients**: 1/2 cup dried elderberries, 1-inch ginger root, 2 cups water, 1/4 cup honey.
- **Method**: Simmer elderberries and ginger in water, strain, cool, and mix with honey. Take 1 tsp daily.
- **Benefits**: Boosts immunity and protects against colds.

14. Warm Lemon and Honey Drink for Colds

- **Ingredients**: Juice of 1/2 lemon, 1 tsp honey, 1 cup warm water.
- **Method**: Mix and drink to soothe sore throats and boost immunity.
- **Benefits**: Hydrates and supports recovery from colds.

15. Cardamom and Ginger Spiced Tea

- **Ingredients**: 3 cardamom pods, 1-inch ginger root, 1 cup water, milk (optional).
- **Method**: Simmer cardamom and ginger in water for 5 minutes, strain, and add milk if desired.
- **Benefits**: Warms the body and aids digestion.

16. Peppermint and Eucalyptus Foot Balm

- **Ingredients**: 2 tbsp coconut oil, 5 drops peppermint essential oil, 5 drops eucalyptus essential oil.
- **Method**: Mix and massage onto feet before bed.
- **Benefits**: Improves circulation and relieves winter aches.

17. Holy Basil (Tulsi) and Ginger Immune Tonic

- **Ingredients**: 1 tsp dried tulsi, 1-inch ginger root, 1 cup boiling water.
- **Method**: Steep tulsi and ginger in boiling water for 10 minutes, strain, and drink.
- **Benefits**: Reduces stress and boosts immunity.

18. Hot Compress with Rosemary and Ginger for Aches

- **Ingredients**: 1 tsp dried rosemary, 1 tsp grated ginger, hot water, clean cloth.

- **Method**: Brew rosemary and ginger in hot water, soak the cloth, and apply to sore areas.
- **Benefits**: Relieves muscle pain and improves circulation.

19. Cinnamon and Nutmeg Milk for Relaxation

- **Ingredients**: 1 cup warm milk, 1/4 tsp cinnamon, a pinch of nutmeg.
- **Method**: Mix and drink warm in the evening.
- **Benefits**: Warms the body and supports restful sleep.

20. Orange Peel and Clove Room Spray

- **Ingredients**: 1/2 cup water, 10 drops orange essential oil, 5 drops clove essential oil.
- **Method**: Mix in a spray bottle and mist around the room.
- **Benefits**: Creates a cozy and uplifting environment.

21. Winter Warming Herb Sachets for Bedding

- **Ingredients**: Dried rosemary, lavender, and cloves, small fabric pouches.
- **Method**: Fill pouches and place under pillows or near bedding.
- **Benefits**: Provides warmth and relaxation for better sleep.

22. Apple and Cinnamon Infused Water

- **Ingredients**: Sliced apple, 1 cinnamon stick, 1 liter warm water.
- **Method**: Combine ingredients in a jug and let steep for 10 minutes.
- **Benefits**: Hydrates and warms the body.

23. Calendula and Beeswax Lip Balm for Winter Cracks

- **Ingredients**: 1/4 cup calendula-infused oil, 1 tbsp beeswax.
- **Method**: Melt beeswax, mix with calendula oil, and store in small jars.
- **Benefits**: Protects and heals dry, cracked lips.

24. Ginger and Mustard Detox Bath

- **Ingredients**: 2 tbsp grated ginger, 1 tbsp mustard powder, warm bathwater.
- **Method**: Add ingredients to the bathwater and soak for 20 minutes.
- **Benefits**: Stimulates circulation and warms the body.

25. Sage and Thyme Gargle for Sore Throats

- **Ingredients**: 1 tsp dried sage, 1 tsp dried thyme, 1 cup hot water.
- **Method**: Steep herbs in hot water for 10 minutes, strain, and gargle 3 times daily.
- **Benefits**: Soothes sore throats and fights infections.

3.10 Emotional Well-Being

Grounding and Stability

1. Holy Basil (Tulsi) Tea for Inner Balance

- **Ingredients**: 1 tsp dried holy basil leaves, 1 cup hot water.
- **Method**: Steep tulsi leaves in hot water for 10 minutes, strain, and drink.
- **Benefits**: Helps to ground emotions and calm a racing mind.

2. Vetiver Essential Oil for Grounding Aromatherapy

- **Ingredients**: 5 drops vetiver essential oil, a diffuser or bowl of hot water.
- **Method**: Add vetiver oil to the diffuser or hot water and inhale deeply for 10 minutes.
- **Benefits**: Creates a sense of stability and calm, especially during chaotic times.

3. Dandelion Root Tea for Emotional Resilience

- **Ingredients**: 1 tsp dried dandelion root, 1 cup boiling water.
- **Method**: Simmer dandelion root in water for 10 minutes, strain, and drink.
- **Benefits**: Encourages emotional release and helps ground feelings of frustration.

4. Mugwort Smudge Stick for Centering Energy

- **Ingredients**: Dried mugwort leaves, cotton string.
- **Method**: Bundle dried mugwort leaves, tie them with string, and burn gently while wafting the smoke around your space.
- **Benefits**: Grounds energy and helps focus scattered thoughts.

5. Chamomile and Oat Infusion for Nervous Stability

- **Ingredients**: 1 tsp dried chamomile flowers, 1 tsp oat straw, 1 cup boiling water.
- **Method**: Steep herbs in boiling water for 10 minutes, strain, and drink.
- **Benefits**: Soothes frayed nerves and promotes emotional stability.

6. Foot Soak with Rosemary and Salt for Grounding

- **Ingredients**: 2 sprigs fresh rosemary, 1/2 cup sea salt, warm water.
- **Method**: Add rosemary and salt to a basin of warm water and soak your feet for 15 minutes.
- **Benefits**: Anchors your energy and promotes physical and emotional grounding.

7. Ashwagandha Root Powder for Emotional Resilience

- **Ingredients**: 1 tsp ashwagandha powder, 1 cup warm milk or plant-based milk.
- **Method**: Mix ashwagandha into the milk and drink at bedtime.
- **Benefits**: Supports adrenal balance and strengthens emotional stability.

8. Frankincense Oil Massage for Calmness

- **Ingredients**: 2 tbsp carrier oil (coconut or almond), 5 drops frankincense essential oil.
- **Method**: Mix oils and massage onto your feet or lower legs before bed.
- **Benefits**: Grounds energy and soothes restlessness.

9. Lemon Balm Tincture for Emotional Stability

- **Ingredients**: 10–15 drops lemon balm tincture in water.
- **Method**: Take twice daily as needed for emotional balance.
- **Benefits**: Reduces nervousness and creates a sense of calm.

10. Yarrow Flower Tea for Strength and Centering

- **Ingredients**: 1 tsp dried yarrow flowers, 1 cup boiling water.
- **Method**: Steep yarrow in boiling water for 10 minutes, strain, and drink.
- **Benefits**: Helps with emotional overwhelm and strengthens boundaries.

11. Cedarwood Essential Oil Diffuser Blend for Stability

- **Ingredients**: 5 drops cedarwood essential oil, diffuser or bowl of hot water.
- **Method**: Add cedarwood oil to the diffuser or hot water and inhale.
- **Benefits**: Grounds emotions and promotes feelings of safety.

12. Grounding Herbal Sachet

- **Ingredients**: Dried lavender, rosemary, and chamomile, small fabric pouch.
- **Method**: Fill the pouch with herbs and keep it in your pocket or near your workspace.
- **Benefits**: Provides subtle, grounding energy throughout the day.

13. Adaptogenic Smoothie for Emotional Stability

- **Ingredients**: 1 tsp maca powder, 1 tsp ashwagandha powder, 1 banana, 1 cup almond milk.
- **Method**: Blend ingredients until smooth and drink as a morning ritual.
- **Benefits**: Supports adrenal health and emotional resilience.

14. Lavender and Sandalwood Bath Soak

- **Ingredients**: 1/2 cup Epsom salt, 5 drops lavender oil, 3 drops sandalwood oil.
- **Method**: Add to warm bathwater and soak for 20 minutes.
- **Benefits**: Grounds the mind and body, easing emotional stress.

15. Valerian Root Tea for Evening Stability

- **Ingredients**: 1 tsp dried valerian root, 1 cup boiling water.
- **Method**: Steep valerian root in boiling water for 10 minutes, strain, and drink before bed.
- **Benefits**: Calms emotional tension and prepares the mind for rest.

16. Grounding Meditation with Sage Tea

- **Ingredients**: 1 tsp dried sage leaves, 1 cup hot water.
- **Method**: Sip slowly while meditating on stability and inner peace.
- **Benefits**: Grounds scattered thoughts and promotes clarity.

17. Licorice Root Tea for Soothing Emotions

- **Ingredients**: 1 tsp dried licorice root, 1 cup boiling water.
- **Method**: Simmer licorice root in water for 10 minutes, strain, and drink.
- **Benefits**: Nourishes the adrenal system and balances emotional highs and lows.

18. Bergamot Oil for Emotional Anchoring

- **Ingredients**: 5 drops bergamot essential oil, diffuser or hot water bowl.
- **Method**: Diffuse or inhale deeply for 10 minutes.
- **Benefits**: Creates emotional balance and lifts a heavy heart.

19. Herbal Incense for Centering

- **Ingredients**: Dried lavender, cedarwood chips, and mugwort.
- **Method**: Burn gently in a safe dish and let the smoke center your energy.
- **Benefits**: Clears mental clutter and grounds your emotions.

20. Ginger and Turmeric Tonic for Stability

- **Ingredients**: 1-inch ginger root, 1/2 tsp turmeric powder, 1 cup water.
- **Method**: Simmer ginger and turmeric in water for 10 minutes, strain, and drink.
- **Benefits**: Boosts circulation and emotional resilience.

21. Skullcap Tea for Nervous Grounding

- **Ingredients**: 1 tsp dried skullcap, 1 cup hot water.
- **Method**: Steep skullcap in hot water for 10 minutes, strain, and drink.
- **Benefits**: Soothes nervous tension and promotes emotional calm.

22. Rose Petal and Honey Infusion for Emotional Warmth

- **Ingredients**: 1 tbsp dried rose petals, 1 tsp honey, 1 cup hot water.
- **Method**: Steep rose petals in water for 10 minutes, strain, and sweeten with honey.
- **Benefits**: Creates emotional comfort and stability.

23. Cinnamon and Cardamom Tea for Emotional Strength

- **Ingredients**: 1 cinnamon stick, 2 cardamom pods, 1 cup hot water.
- **Method**: Simmer spices in water for 10 minutes, strain, and drink.
- **Benefits**: Warms and stabilizes the body and emotions.

24. Herbal Poultice for Heart-Centered Stability

- **Ingredients**: Fresh rose petals and lavender flowers, a clean cloth.
- **Method**: Crush petals and flowers, wrap in cloth, and place over the heart for 15 minutes.
- **Benefits**: Soothes emotional unrest and encourages self-love.

25. Myrrh Oil for Deep Stability

- **Ingredients**: 5 drops myrrh essential oil, diffuser or bowl of warm water.
- **Method**: Inhale deeply for 10 minutes.
- **Benefits**: Grounds deep emotional instability and promotes spiritual connection.

Emotional Detox and Release

1. Rose and Lavender Bath for Emotional Cleansing

- **Ingredients**: 1/2 cup dried rose petals, 1/4 cup dried lavender, warm bathwater.
- **Method**: Add rose petals and lavender to the bathwater, soak for 20 minutes.
- **Benefits**: Helps release sadness and promotes emotional balance.

2. Hawthorn Berry Tea for Letting Go

- **Ingredients**: 1 tsp dried hawthorn berries, 1 cup boiling water.
- **Method**: Steep berries in hot water for 15 minutes, strain, and drink.
- **Benefits**: Supports the emotional heart and helps process grief.

3. Lemon Balm Tincture for Emotional Clarity

- **Ingredients**: 10–15 drops lemon balm tincture in water.
- **Method**: Take once or twice daily when feeling overwhelmed.
- **Benefits**: Calms the mind and promotes emotional clarity.

4. Skullcap Tea for Releasing Emotional Tension

- **Ingredients**: 1 tsp dried skullcap, 1 cup boiling water.
- **Method**: Steep for 10 minutes, strain, and drink.
- **Benefits**: Soothes nervous tension and aids in emotional release.

5. Jasmine Essential Oil for Releasing Heartache

- **Ingredients**: 5 drops jasmine essential oil, diffuser or cotton pad.
- **Method**: Diffuse or inhale deeply for 10 minutes.
- **Benefits**: Opens the heart and encourages the release of pent-up emotions.

6. Chamomile and Rose Petal Compress

- **Ingredients**: 1 tbsp dried chamomile, 1 tbsp dried rose petals, hot water, clean cloth.
- **Method**: Brew herbs in hot water, soak the cloth, and place it over the chest for 15 minutes.
- **Benefits**: Helps release emotional heaviness and calms the heart.

7. Herbal Journaling Ritual with Holy Basil Tea

- **Ingredients**: 1 tsp dried holy basil, 1 cup boiling water.
- **Method**: Brew tea and sip while journaling about your emotions.
- **Benefits**: Creates a safe space for emotional detox and reflection.

8. Lavender and Bergamot Aromatherapy for Inner Peace

- **Ingredients**: 5 drops lavender essential oil, 5 drops bergamot essential oil.
- **Method**: Diffuse oils in your space or add to a warm compress.
- **Benefits**: Encourages emotional release and balances energy.

9. Calendula Salve for Nurturing Self-Compassion

- **Ingredients**: 1/4 cup calendula-infused oil, 1 tbsp beeswax.
- **Method**: Melt beeswax, mix with calendula oil, and apply to hands or heart area.
- **Benefits**: Promotes self-love and emotional comfort.

10. Passionflower Tea for Emotional Release

- **Ingredients**: 1 tsp dried passionflower, 1 cup boiling water.
- **Method**: Steep for 10 minutes, strain, and drink.
- **Benefits**: Helps process intense emotions and releases emotional tension.

11. Sage Smudging for Clearing Emotional Energy

- **Ingredients**: A sage smudge stick.
- **Method**: Light the smudge stick and waft the smoke around your body or space.
- **Benefits**: Clears lingering emotional energy and creates a fresh start.

12. Herbal Detox Foot Soak

- **Ingredients**: 1/2 cup Epsom salt, 1 tbsp dried rosemary, warm water.
- **Method**: Add ingredients to a basin and soak feet for 15 minutes.
- **Benefits**: Releases emotional blockages and promotes grounding.

13. Lemon and Ginger Infusion for Emotional Renewal

- **Ingredients**: 1 slice fresh ginger, juice of 1/2 lemon, 1 cup boiling water.

- **Method**: Steep for 10 minutes, strain, and drink.
- **Benefits**: Detoxifies and energizes the emotional body.

14. Dandelion Root Tea for Letting Go of Resentment

- **Ingredients**: 1 tsp dried dandelion root, 1 cup water.
- **Method**: Simmer root in water for 10 minutes, strain, and drink.
- **Benefits**: Supports emotional detox and releases stagnant feelings.

15. Rosehip and Hibiscus Tea for Emotional Renewal

- **Ingredients**: 1 tsp dried rosehips, 1 tsp dried hibiscus, 1 cup boiling water.
- **Method**: Steep for 10 minutes, strain, and drink.
- **Benefits**: Refreshes the emotional spirit and provides vitamin C for renewal.

16. Lavender Pillow Spray for Dream Release

- **Ingredients**: 1/2 cup distilled water, 10 drops lavender essential oil, spray bottle.
- **Method**: Mix in a spray bottle and spritz onto your pillow before sleep.
- **Benefits**: Encourages emotional processing during restful sleep.

17. Fennel Seed Tea for Digestive and Emotional Release

- **Ingredients**: 1 tsp fennel seeds, 1 cup boiling water.
- **Method**: Steep for 10 minutes, strain, and drink.
- **Benefits**: Aids digestion and helps release emotions stored in the gut.

18. Ylang-Ylang Oil for Emotional Healing

- **Ingredients**: 5 drops ylang-ylang essential oil, carrier oil for massage.
- **Method**: Mix and massage onto the wrists or chest.
- **Benefits**: Helps process grief and promotes emotional healing.

19. Valerian Root Tea for Deep Release

- **Ingredients**: 1 tsp dried valerian root, 1 cup boiling water.
- **Method**: Steep for 10 minutes, strain, and drink before bed.
- **Benefits**: Supports emotional release through deep relaxation.

20. Peppermint and Lemon Foot Compress

- **Ingredients**: 1 tsp dried peppermint, 1 tsp dried lemon balm, warm water, clean cloth.
- **Method**: Brew herbs in water, soak the cloth, and place on feet.
- **Benefits**: Refreshes the mind and helps release pent-up emotions.

21. Neroli and Rose Facial Steam for Emotional Comfort

- **Ingredients**: 5 drops neroli oil, 5 drops rose oil, bowl of hot water.
- **Method**: Add oils to the bowl, cover your head with a towel, and steam your face for 10 minutes.
- **Benefits**: Eases sadness and promotes emotional softness.

22. Mugwort Tea for Processing Emotions

- **Ingredients**: 1 tsp dried mugwort, 1 cup boiling water.
- **Method**: Steep for 10 minutes, strain, and drink.
- **Benefits**: Helps access and process deeper emotions.

23. Ginger and Cinnamon Tonic for Emotional Warmth

- **Ingredients**: 1-inch ginger root, 1 cinnamon stick, 1 cup water.
- **Method**: Simmer ginger and cinnamon in water for 10 minutes, strain, and drink.
- **Benefits**: Warms the emotional body and supports release.

24. Bergamot and Chamomile Diffuser Blend

- **Ingredients**: 5 drops bergamot oil, 5 drops chamomile oil, diffuser.
- **Method**: Add to a diffuser and run in your space.
- **Benefits**: Lifts heavy emotions and promotes peace.

25. Rosemary Infused Hair Rinse for Emotional Detox

- **Ingredients**: 1/4 cup dried rosemary, 1 cup boiling water.
- **Method**: Steep rosemary in boiling water, cool, and use as a final hair rinse.
- **Benefits**: Symbolically washes away emotional residue and refreshes the mind.

Joy and Positivity

1. Citrus and Mint Uplifting Tea

- **Ingredients**: 1 tsp dried orange peel, 1 tsp dried peppermint leaves, 1 cup hot water.
- **Method**: Steep the herbs in hot water for 10 minutes, strain, and drink.
- **Benefits**: Energizes the mind and creates a bright, cheerful mood.

2. Lemon Balm and Honey Morning Ritual

- **Ingredients**: 1 tsp dried lemon balm, 1 cup hot water, 1 tsp honey.
- **Method**: Brew tea, sweeten with honey, and enjoy as part of a calm, reflective morning routine.
- **Benefits**: Promotes optimism and clears mental fog.

3. Orange and Bergamot Diffuser Blend

- **Ingredients**: 5 drops orange essential oil, 5 drops bergamot essential oil, water for diffuser.
- **Method**: Add oils to a diffuser and let the scent fill the room.
- **Benefits**: Lifts a heavy heart and fosters an atmosphere of joy.

4. Calendula Flower Infusion for Emotional Warmth

- **Ingredients**: 1 tbsp dried calendula petals, 1 cup boiling water.
- **Method**: Steep calendula in boiling water for 10 minutes, strain, and drink.
- **Benefits**: Symbolically represents sunshine and joy, promoting emotional warmth.

5. Herbal Gratitude Journal Practice

- **Ingredients**: 1 cup chamomile or rose tea (optional).
- **Method**: While sipping tea, write three things you're grateful for daily.
- **Benefits**: Combines herbs with mindfulness to nurture positivity.

6. Nature Walk for Emotional Renewal

- **Practice**: Take a slow, mindful walk in nature, focusing on the sights, sounds, and smells around you.
- **Benefits**: Reconnects with nature's rhythms, boosts serotonin, and promotes inner joy.

7. St. John's Wort Tea for Emotional Brightness

- **Ingredients**: 1 tsp dried St. John's Wort, 1 cup boiling water.
- **Method**: Steep for 10 minutes, strain, and drink.

- **Benefits**: Naturally boosts mood and helps manage seasonal sadness.

8. Lemon and Rosemary Hand Scrub

- **Ingredients**: 2 tbsp sugar, 1 tbsp olive oil, 5 drops lemon essential oil, 5 drops rosemary essential oil.
- **Method**: Mix ingredients and massage onto hands, then rinse.
- **Benefits**: Uplifts the senses and provides a moment of joyful self-care.

9. Lavender and Peppermint Foot Soak

- **Ingredients**: 1/4 cup Epsom salt, 5 drops lavender essential oil, 5 drops peppermint essential oil, warm water.
- **Method**: Add to a basin and soak feet for 15 minutes.
- **Benefits**: Revitalizes tired feet and refreshes the mind.

10. Citrus Fruit Bowl for Visual Joy

- **Practice**: Keep a bowl of vibrant citrus fruits (lemons, oranges, grapefruits) in your kitchen or living space.
- **Benefits**: The bright colors and natural aromas stimulate joy and energy.

11. Sun-Gazing for Positivity

- **Practice**: Spend 5–10 minutes outdoors during sunrise or sunset, letting the sunlight gently fall on your face (avoid direct midday sun).
- **Benefits**: Improves mood by stimulating serotonin production.

12. Rose and Hibiscus Body Mist

- **Ingredients**: 1/2 cup rosewater, 1/4 cup hibiscus infusion, spray bottle.
- **Method**: Mix and spritz lightly onto skin throughout the day.
- **Benefits**: Hydrates the skin and creates a refreshing, joyful aura.

13. Lemon Verbena Pillow Sachets for Happy Dreams

- **Ingredients**: Dried lemon verbena, small fabric pouches.
- **Method**: Fill the pouches with dried herb and place under your pillow.
- **Benefits**: Promotes positive dreams and lightens the spirit.

14. Morning Peppermint and Rosemary Shower

- **Practice**: Hang fresh rosemary and peppermint sprigs in your shower to release their aromas with the steam.
- **Benefits**: Stimulates the senses and starts the day on a joyful note.

15. Ginger and Turmeric Mood-Boosting Latte

- **Ingredients**: 1/2 tsp turmeric, 1/4 tsp ginger powder, 1 cup warm milk, 1 tsp honey.
- **Method**: Mix all ingredients and drink warm.
- **Benefits**: Enhances emotional energy and creates inner warmth.

16. Fresh Flower Arrangement for Emotional Brightness

- **Practice**: Arrange fresh, colorful flowers in your living space.
- **Benefits**: Adds beauty and joy to your environment.

17. Holy Basil and Lemongrass Positivity Tea

- **Ingredients**: 1 tsp holy basil, 1 tsp dried lemongrass, 1 cup boiling water.
- **Method**: Steep for 10 minutes, strain, and drink.
- **Benefits**: Balances emotions and creates mental clarity.

18. Evening Sky Watching for Awe and Joy

- **Practice**: Spend time looking at the stars or sunset, reflecting on the beauty of the universe.
- **Benefits**: Cultivates gratitude and a sense of wonder.

19. Citrus and Lavender Body Oil

- **Ingredients**: 2 tbsp carrier oil, 5 drops orange essential oil, 3 drops lavender essential oil.
- **Method**: Mix and massage onto skin after a shower.
- **Benefits**: Refreshes the body and uplifts the spirit.

20. Peppermint and Lemon Balm Mood Tea

- **Ingredients**: 1 tsp dried peppermint, 1 tsp dried lemon balm, 1 cup boiling water.
- **Method**: Steep for 10 minutes, strain, and drink.
- **Benefits**: Soothes the nerves and promotes light-heartedness.

21. Walking Barefoot on Grass (Earthing)

- **Practice**: Spend a few minutes walking barefoot on grass, focusing on the sensation.
- **Benefits**: Grounds the body and mind, releasing tension and promoting joy.

22. Vanilla and Cinnamon Room Spray

- **Ingredients**: 1/2 cup water, 5 drops vanilla extract, 1/4 tsp cinnamon oil.
- **Method**: Mix in a spray bottle and mist your room.
- **Benefits**: Creates a cozy, joyful environment.

23. Gratitude Walk with Aromatic Herbs

- **Practice**: Carry a small sprig of rosemary or mint on a walk, inhaling its scent while mentally listing things you're grateful for.
- **Benefits**: Combines movement, mindfulness, and herbs to spark joy.

24. Herbal Potpourri for Joyful Spaces

- **Ingredients**: Dried orange slices, cinnamon sticks, cloves, and lavender.
- **Method**: Mix ingredients and place in a decorative bowl.
- **Benefits**: Fills the room with uplifting scents.

25. Lemon Balm and Rose Petal Water for Positivity

- **Ingredients**: 1 tsp dried lemon balm, 1 tsp dried rose petals, 1 cup boiling water.
- **Method**: Brew as tea or use as a facial rinse.
- **Benefits**: Refreshes the spirit and skin, bringing lightness and joy.

Self-Love and Compassion

1. Rose Petal and Honey Infusion for Heart Healing

- **Ingredients**: 1 tbsp dried rose petals, 1 tsp honey, 1 cup boiling water.
- **Method**: Steep rose petals in boiling water for 10 minutes, strain, and sweeten with honey.
- **Benefits**: Encourages emotional warmth and promotes self-compassion.

2. Lavender and Vanilla Aromatherapy Bath

- **Ingredients**: 1/2 cup Epsom salt, 5 drops lavender essential oil, 1/4 tsp vanilla extract.
- **Method**: Add to warm bathwater and soak for 20 minutes.
- **Benefits**: Relaxes the body, soothes the mind, and creates space for self-care.

3. Herbal Affirmation Ritual with Chamomile Tea

- **Ingredients**: 1 tsp dried chamomile flowers, 1 cup boiling water.
- **Method**: While sipping chamomile tea, recite positive affirmations like, "I am enough," or "I am worthy of love."
- **Benefits**: Combines herbal calming effects with self-affirming words.

4. Holy Basil Tea for Emotional Centering

- **Ingredients**: 1 tsp dried holy basil, 1 cup hot water.
- **Method**: Steep for 10 minutes, strain, and drink during quiet reflection.
- **Benefits**: Grounds emotions and fosters self-awareness.

5. Self-Massage with Calendula Oil

- **Ingredients**: 2 tbsp calendula-infused oil, 5 drops frankincense essential oil.
- **Method**: Warm oil and massage onto your arms, hands, or feet while focusing on gratitude for your body.
- **Benefits**: Promotes self-connection and nourishes the skin.

6. Gratitude Journal with Lavender-Infused Water

- **Ingredients**: 1/4 cup dried lavender, 2 cups boiling water.
- **Method**: Steep lavender, strain, and use as a calming drink while journaling about things you love about yourself.
- **Benefits**: Combines emotional reflection with herbal soothing.

7. Rose Quartz and Herbal Bath Ritual

- **Ingredients**: Dried rose petals, lavender buds, and a rose quartz crystal.
- **Method**: Place herbs and rose quartz in warm bathwater and soak while focusing on self-love intentions.
- **Benefits**: Symbolically infuses your bath with love and emotional healing.

8. Jasmine Tea for Inner Nurturing

- **Ingredients**: 1 tsp dried jasmine flowers, 1 cup hot water.
- **Method**: Steep for 5–10 minutes, strain, and drink during a moment of solitude.
- **Benefits**: Encourages emotional softness and connection to oneself.

9. Peppermint and Lemon Balm Foot Soak

- **Ingredients**: 1/4 cup Epsom salt, 5 drops peppermint essential oil, 1 tsp dried lemon balm, warm water.
- **Method**: Add ingredients to a basin and soak feet for 15 minutes.
- **Benefits**: Refreshes the body and creates a ritual of self-kindness.

10. Morning Rosemary and Orange Essential Oil Ritual

- **Ingredients**: 5 drops rosemary essential oil, 5 drops orange essential oil, diffuser.
- **Method**: Diffuse oils while preparing for the day, repeating affirmations like, "Today, I choose love and kindness toward myself."
- **Benefits**: Energizes and centers the mind with positivity.

11. Sacred Space with Herbal Incense

- **Ingredients**: Dried lavender, rosemary, and sage.
- **Method**: Burn herbs as incense to create a sacred space for self-reflection or meditation.
- **Benefits**: Clears mental clutter and promotes emotional clarity.

12. Mugwort and Chamomile Dream Pillow

- **Ingredients**: Dried mugwort, chamomile, and a small fabric pouch.
- **Method**: Fill the pouch with herbs and place under your pillow to inspire restful, self-reflective dreams.
- **Benefits**: Encourages subconscious processing and emotional release.

13. Gratitude Walk with Holy Basil Tea

- **Practice**: Sip holy basil tea before taking a walk, focusing on things you appreciate about yourself and your surroundings.
- **Benefits**: Combines mindfulness, movement, and herbs for emotional renewal.

14. Self-Compassion Facial with Aloe and Lavender Oil

- **Ingredients**: 1 tbsp aloe vera gel, 2 drops lavender essential oil.
- **Method**: Mix and apply to your face as a mask, leaving it on for 10 minutes.
- **Benefits**: Hydrates the skin and creates a nurturing ritual of self-care.

15. Lemon Balm and Peppermint Positivity Tea

- **Ingredients**: 1 tsp dried lemon balm, 1 tsp dried peppermint, 1 cup hot water.
- **Method**: Steep for 10 minutes, strain, and drink while focusing on joy.
- **Benefits**: Lifts the spirit and encourages a positive outlook.

16. Journaling with Lavender-Infused Candles

- **Practice**: Light a lavender-scented candle and journal about acts of kindness you've shown yourself recently.
- **Benefits**: Cultivates gratitude and compassion for oneself.

17. Calendula and Rose Petal Body Scrub

- **Ingredients**: 1/4 cup sugar, 1 tbsp dried calendula petals, 1 tbsp dried rose petals, 2 tbsp coconut oil.
- **Method**: Blend into a scrub and massage onto the skin during a shower.
- **Benefits**: Gently exfoliates and symbolizes emotional renewal.

18. Sunlight Meditation for Radiance

- **Practice**: Sit in a sunny spot for 10 minutes, visualizing light filling your body with warmth and self-love.
- **Benefits**: Energizes the body and fosters positive emotions.

19. Sandalwood and Rosewater Face Mist

- **Ingredients**: 1/2 cup rosewater, 5 drops sandalwood essential oil, spray bottle.
- **Method**: Mix and spritz on your face or around your space.
- **Benefits**: Creates a calming, loving environment for self-care.

20. Valerian Root Tea for Deep Relaxation

- **Ingredients**: 1 tsp dried valerian root, 1 cup hot water.
- **Method**: Steep for 10 minutes, strain, and drink before bed.
- **Benefits**: Encourages restful sleep and supports emotional recovery.

21. Walking Meditation with Lavender Hand Oil

- **Ingredients**: 1 tbsp coconut oil, 5 drops lavender essential oil.
- **Method**: Massage onto hands before taking a meditative walk, focusing on your breath and surroundings.
- **Benefits**: Combines movement and touch for deep relaxation.

22. Adaptogen Smoothie for Inner Resilience

- **Ingredients**: 1 tsp ashwagandha powder, 1 banana, 1 cup almond milk.
- **Method**: Blend and enjoy as a nourishing self-care ritual.
- **Benefits**: Builds resilience and supports emotional strength.

23. Evening Lavender and Peppermint Aromatherapy

- **Ingredients**: 3 drops lavender oil, 2 drops peppermint oil, diffuser.
- **Method**: Diffuse oils during evening self-reflection time.
- **Benefits**: Calms the mind and promotes clarity.

24. Lemon Balm and Rose Tea for Heart-Centered Reflection

- **Ingredients**: 1 tsp lemon balm, 1 tsp dried rose petals, 1 cup hot water.
- **Method**: Steep for 10 minutes, strain, and drink during journaling or meditation.
- **Benefits**: Opens the heart and supports emotional healing.

25. Gratitude Bath with Fresh Flowers

- **Ingredients**: Fresh flowers (roses, lavender, chamomile), warm bathwater.
- **Method**: Float flowers in the bath and soak while reflecting on acts of kindness you've shown yourself.
- **Benefits**: A symbolic and sensory ritual for cultivating self-love.

3.11 Longevity And Spiritual Growth

Sustaining Life's Flame

1. Ginseng Energy Tonic

- **Ingredients**: 1 tsp ginseng root (dried or powdered), 1 cup hot water.
- **Method**: Simmer ginseng in hot water for 10 minutes, strain, and drink in the morning.
- **Benefits**: Boosts stamina, energy levels, and endurance.

2. Ashwagandha Nighttime Restorative Milk

- **Ingredients**: 1 tsp ashwagandha powder, 1 cup warm milk, 1/4 tsp cinnamon, 1 tsp honey.
- **Method**: Mix ashwagandha powder into warm milk, add cinnamon and honey, and drink before bed.
- **Benefits**: Supports adrenal health and replenishes energy reserves during rest.

3. Adaptogenic Morning Smoothie

- **Ingredients**: 1 tsp maca powder, 1 tsp schisandra berry powder, 1 banana, 1 cup almond milk.
- **Method**: Blend ingredients until smooth and enjoy as a breakfast ritual.
- **Benefits**: Enhances vitality and balances the body's stress response.

4. Nettle Infusion for Daily Vitality

- **Ingredients**: 1 tbsp dried nettle leaves, 1 cup boiling water.
- **Method**: Steep nettle leaves in boiling water for 10 minutes, strain, and drink.
- **Benefits**: Provides a rich source of minerals and supports energy production.

5. Cordyceps Mushroom Tonic for Endurance

- **Ingredients**: 1 tsp cordyceps powder, 1 cup hot water.
- **Method**: Steep cordyceps powder in hot water for 10 minutes and drink.
- **Benefits**: Enhances physical stamina and supports lung health.

6. Seasonal Ritual: Spring Vitality Tonic

- **Ingredients**: 1 tsp dandelion root, 1 tsp burdock root, 1 cup water.
- **Method**: Simmer herbs in water for 10 minutes, strain, and drink.
- **Benefits**: Detoxifies and revitalizes the body during seasonal transitions.

7. Lemon Balm Tea for Gentle Energy

- **Ingredients**: 1 tsp dried lemon balm, 1 cup boiling water.
- **Method**: Steep for 10 minutes, strain, and drink as a mid-afternoon pick-me-up.
- **Benefits**: Calms the mind while promoting a steady flow of energy.

8. Holy Basil (Tulsi) and Ginger Tea

- **Ingredients**: 1 tsp dried holy basil, 1 tsp grated ginger, 1 cup boiling water.
- **Method**: Steep holy basil and ginger in hot water for 10 minutes, strain, and drink.
- **Benefits**: Balances energy and supports the body's natural rhythms.

9. Astragalus Root Soup for Immunity and Energy

- **Ingredients**: 2–3 slices of astragalus root, vegetable broth, and seasonal vegetables.
- **Method**: Simmer astragalus root in the broth for 30 minutes, add vegetables, and enjoy.
- **Benefits**: Boosts immune function and maintains energy levels.

10. Reishi Mushroom Tea for Inner Balance

- **Ingredients**: 1 tsp reishi mushroom powder, 1 cup hot water.
- **Method**: Steep reishi powder in hot water for 15 minutes, strain, and drink in the evening.
- **Benefits**: Supports energy restoration and promotes spiritual grounding.

11. Herbal Hydration Water

- **Ingredients**: 1 cucumber slice, 1 sprig mint, 1 tsp dried hibiscus, 1 liter water.
- **Method**: Infuse ingredients in water for 2–3 hours and drink throughout the day.
- **Benefits**: Hydrates and gently energizes the body.

12. Morning Qi-Gong with Herbal Tea

- **Practice**: Drink holy basil tea before practicing gentle qi-gong movements to awaken and balance life energy.
- **Benefits**: Strengthens vital energy and aligns the body with nature's flow.

13. Schisandra Berry Infusion for Resilience

- **Ingredients**: 1 tsp dried schisandra berries, 1 cup boiling water.
- **Method**: Steep for 10 minutes, strain, and drink.
- **Benefits**: Balances stress response and enhances resilience.

14. Ginkgo Biloba Tea for Circulation

- **Ingredients**: 1 tsp dried ginkgo leaves, 1 cup boiling water.
- **Method**: Steep for 10 minutes, strain, and drink.
- **Benefits**: Improves circulation and enhances energy delivery to the brain and body.

15. Cinnamon and Honey Elixir

- **Ingredients**: 1/2 tsp cinnamon powder, 1 tsp raw honey, 1 cup warm water.
- **Method**: Mix and drink first thing in the morning.
- **Benefits**: Provides an energizing start to the day and supports metabolism.

16. Rhodiola Energy Tonic

- **Ingredients**: 1 tsp rhodiola root powder, 1 cup hot water.
- **Method**: Steep rhodiola in hot water for 10 minutes, strain, and drink in the morning.
- **Benefits**: Enhances endurance and reduces fatigue.

17. Herb-Infused Oil for Vitality Massage

- **Ingredients**: 1/4 cup olive oil, 1 tsp dried rosemary, 1 tsp dried ginger.
- **Method**: Infuse herbs in oil for 2 weeks, strain, and use for self-massage.
- **Benefits**: Improves circulation and energizes the body.

18. Golden Milk with Turmeric and Ashwagandha

- **Ingredients**: 1/2 tsp turmeric, 1/2 tsp ashwagandha powder, 1 cup warm milk, 1 tsp honey.
- **Method**: Mix ingredients and drink at night.
- **Benefits**: Restores energy while reducing inflammation.

19. Herb-Infused Sauna Ritual

- **Ingredients**: 1 sprig rosemary, 1 tsp lavender flowers.

- **Method**: Add herbs to a steam room or sauna session for aromatherapy.
- **Benefits**: Opens pores and energizes the body through herbal steam.

20. Energizing Breathing Ritual with Mint Tea

- **Practice**: Sip mint tea and practice deep, rhythmic breathing to stimulate energy flow.
- **Benefits**: Combines physical and mental rejuvenation.

21. Apple Cider Vinegar and Honey Tonic

- **Ingredients**: 1 tbsp apple cider vinegar, 1 tsp honey, 1 cup warm water.
- **Method**: Mix and drink in the morning.
- **Benefits**: Balances pH levels and supports sustained energy.

22. Black Sesame Seed Paste for Longevity

- **Ingredients**: 1/4 cup black sesame seeds, 1 tsp honey.
- **Method**: Grind sesame seeds into a paste, mix with honey, and eat 1 tsp daily.
- **Benefits**: Nourishes energy and supports kidney health in traditional practices.

23. Morning Sun Ritual with Herbal Tea

- **Practice**: Enjoy holy basil or nettle tea while sitting in the morning sunlight for 10 minutes.
- **Benefits**: Boosts vitamin D, energizes the body, and aligns with nature.

24. Herbal Soup with Ginger and Turmeric

- **Ingredients**: 1 tsp grated ginger, 1/2 tsp turmeric powder, vegetable broth.
- **Method**: Simmer ingredients and enjoy as a warming meal.
- **Benefits**: Combats fatigue and restores energy.

25. Evening Reflection with Lemon Balm Tea

- **Ingredients**: 1 tsp dried lemon balm, 1 cup hot water.
- **Method**: Steep for 10 minutes, strain, and drink while journaling.
- **Benefits**: Calms the mind while promoting inner energy for the next day.

Renewal and Inner Radiance

1. Rose and Holy Basil (Tulsi) Tea for Heart Renewal

- **Ingredients**: 1 tsp dried rose petals, 1 tsp holy basil, 1 cup boiling water.
- **Method**: Steep for 10 minutes, strain, and drink while reflecting on self-love and compassion.
- **Benefits**: Opens the heart chakra and fosters emotional renewal.

2. Lavender and Frankincense Sacred Meditation Oil

- **Ingredients**: 5 drops lavender essential oil, 3 drops frankincense essential oil, 2 tbsp carrier oil.
- **Method**: Mix and anoint your pulse points before meditation.
- **Benefits**: Creates spiritual calm and enhances mindfulness practices.

3. Gratitude Ritual with Lemon Balm Tea

- **Ingredients**: 1 tsp dried lemon balm, 1 cup boiling water.
- **Method**: Sip the tea while journaling three things you're grateful for each day.
- **Benefits**: Grounds the spirit and cultivates inner radiance through gratitude.

4. Mugwort Dreamwork Ritual

- **Ingredients**: 1 tsp dried mugwort, 1 cup boiling water.
- **Method**: Steep for 10 minutes, strain, and sip before sleep. Reflect on your dreams upon waking.
- **Benefits**: Enhances spiritual insight and connects you with the subconscious.

5. Reishi Mushroom Tea for Inner Strength

- **Ingredients**: 1 tsp reishi mushroom powder, 1 cup hot water.
- **Method**: Brew and drink during moments of reflection or after prayer.
- **Benefits**: Builds spiritual resilience and nourishes the spirit.

6. Herbal Cleansing Bath for Renewal

- **Ingredients**: 1/4 cup dried rosemary, 1/4 cup dried sage, 1/4 cup Epsom salt.
- **Method**: Add to warm bathwater and soak for 20 minutes, focusing on letting go of emotional baggage.
- **Benefits**: Cleanses the energetic field and restores spiritual clarity.

7. Rose and Sandalwood Smudging Ritual

- **Ingredients**: Dried rose petals, a pinch of sandalwood powder, smudge stick or charcoal disc.
- **Method**: Burn gently and waft the smoke over yourself or your space.
- **Benefits**: Invites love, peace, and inner harmony into your environment.

8. Guided Meditation with Holy Basil Tea

- **Ingredients**: 1 tsp dried holy basil, 1 cup boiling water.
- **Method**: Brew and sip tea before a guided meditation session.
- **Benefits**: Centers the spirit and fosters spiritual connection.

9. Journaling with Sacred Herbs

- **Practice**: Light incense with frankincense and sandalwood, and write about your intentions or spiritual growth.
- **Benefits**: Enhances clarity and deepens the connection with your inner self.

10. Morning Sun Salutation with Adaptogenic Tea

- **Ingredients**: 1 tsp ashwagandha powder, 1 cup hot water.
- **Method**: Drink after a few sun salutations, focusing on your connection to the natural world.
- **Benefits**: Grounds and energizes the body and mind.

11. Chakra Balancing with Herbs

- **Practice**: Use specific herbs for each chakra. For example, peppermint for the throat chakra (communication) or chamomile for the solar plexus (confidence).
- **Benefits**: Restores energetic balance and fosters spiritual vitality.

12. Spiritual Fasting with Herbal Water

- **Ingredients**: 1 liter water, 1 tsp fresh mint leaves, 1 slice cucumber, and a squeeze of lemon.
- **Method**: Drink throughout a day of intentional fasting and reflection.
- **Benefits**: Supports clarity, focus, and spiritual renewal.

13. Evening Rose and Lavender Tea for Renewal

- **Ingredients**: 1 tsp dried rose petals, 1 tsp dried lavender, 1 cup boiling water.
- **Method**: Steep and sip while reflecting on your day.

- **Benefits**: Calms the mind and soothes the spirit, fostering renewal.

14. Sacred Space Cleansing with Sage and Mugwort

- **Ingredients**: 1 sage smudge stick, a small bundle of dried mugwort.
- **Method**: Burn and use the smoke to cleanse a space for meditation or spiritual work.
- **Benefits**: Removes stagnant energy and invites clarity.

15. Sound Healing with Herbal Tea

- **Practice**: Pair sound healing (e.g., Tibetan singing bowls or chimes) with holy basil or chamomile tea.
- **Benefits**: Aligns the body and spirit, releasing tension and renewing energy.

16. Sandalwood Candle Meditation

- **Ingredients**: Sandalwood-scented candle.
- **Method**: Light the candle, focus on the flame, and repeat affirmations of renewal and strength.
- **Benefits**: Fosters peace and spiritual rejuvenation.

17. Adaptogen-Infused Yoga Practice

- **Ingredients**: 1 tsp schisandra berry powder, 1 cup hot water.
- **Method**: Sip before practicing gentle yoga poses.
- **Benefits**: Supports stamina and enhances connection with the body.

18. Visualization with Lemon Balm and Mint Tea

- **Ingredients**: 1 tsp dried lemon balm, 1 tsp dried mint, 1 cup hot water.
- **Method**: Sip while visualizing a future full of purpose and joy.
- **Benefits**: Combines mindfulness and herbal support to inspire renewal.

19. Gratitude Stones with Sacred Herbs

- **Practice**: Hold a stone (like rose quartz) while burning lavender incense. Reflect on what you're grateful for.
- **Benefits**: Cultivates a radiant spirit through gratitude.

20. Fennel and Ginger Infusion for Release

- **Ingredients**: 1 tsp fennel seeds, 1 slice ginger, 1 cup boiling water.
- **Method**: Steep and sip during emotional release practices, such as journaling.
- **Benefits**: Releases stuck energy and promotes emotional cleansing.

21. Moon Ritual with Herbal Tea

- **Practice**: During a full moon, sip chamomile or lavender tea while journaling intentions for renewal.
- **Benefits**: Aligns your spiritual cycle with nature's rhythms.

22. Breathing Ritual with Vetiver Oil

- **Ingredients**: 2 drops vetiver essential oil.
- **Method**: Place a drop on your wrists and practice deep breathing for 5 minutes.
- **Benefits**: Grounds the spirit and calms emotional energy.

23. Self-Compassion Tea Ceremony

- **Ingredients**: 1 tsp dried rose petals, 1 tsp lemon balm, 1 cup hot water.
- **Method**: Sip the tea while reciting affirmations like, "I am worthy of love and renewal."
- **Benefits**: Nurtures the heart and fosters spiritual connection.

24. Energy Detox with Rosemary Tea

- **Ingredients**: 1 tsp dried rosemary, 1 cup boiling water.
- **Method**: Steep for 10 minutes, strain, and drink. Reflect on releasing negative energy.
- **Benefits**: Cleanses the spirit and refreshes the mind.

25. Prayer with Jasmine and Rose Incense

- **Ingredients**: Jasmine and rose incense sticks.
- **Method**: Burn incense during moments of prayer or spiritual reflection.
- **Benefits**: Enhances spiritual connection and fosters inner peace.

Deepening Meditation & Mindfulness

1. Frankincense and Sandalwood Meditation Incense

- **Ingredients:** 1 tsp powdered frankincense, 1 tsp powdered sandalwood, charcoal disc.
- **Method:** Burn the blend on a charcoal disc during meditation.
- **Benefits:** Deepens spiritual focus and calms the mind.

2. Holy Basil (Tulsi) Tea for Centering

- **Ingredients:** 1 tsp dried holy basil leaves, 1 cup boiling water.
- **Method:** Steep for 10 minutes, strain, and drink before meditation.
- **Benefits:** Enhances emotional balance and prepares the mind for mindfulness.

3. Lavender and Peppermint Mindfulness Spray

- **Ingredients**: 1/2 cup distilled water, 5 drops lavender oil, 5 drops peppermint oil, spray bottle.
- **Method**: Mix in a spray bottle and mist the air around your meditation space.
- **Benefits**: Promotes relaxation and mental clarity.

4. Mugwort and Sage Cleansing Ritual

- **Ingredients**: 1 dried mugwort bundle, 1 sage smudge stick.
- **Method**: Light the smudge sticks and waft the smoke around your body or space before meditation.
- **Benefits**: Clears stagnant energy and prepares the spirit for reflection.

5. Chamomile and Lemon Balm Calming Tea

- **Ingredients**: 1 tsp dried chamomile, 1 tsp dried lemon balm, 1 cup boiling water.
- **Method**: Steep for 10 minutes, strain, and sip slowly.
- **Benefits**: Soothes the nervous system and reduces distractions.

6. Guided Visualization with Rose Tea

- **Ingredients**: 1 tsp dried rose petals, 1 cup boiling water.
- **Method**: Brew tea and drink while practicing a guided visualization (e.g., envisioning a peaceful garden).
- **Benefits**: Enhances imagination and creates a peaceful mental space.

7. Morning Breathing Ritual with Mint Tea

- **Ingredients**: 1 tsp dried mint leaves, 1 cup boiling water.
- **Method**: Sip mint tea while practicing 10 minutes of deep belly breathing.
- **Benefits**: Clears mental fog and energizes the mind for meditation.

8. Meditation Candle with Essential Oils

- **Ingredients**: Unscented candle, 2 drops sandalwood oil, 2 drops lavender oil.
- **Method**: Add essential oils to the candle before lighting it for meditation.
- **Benefits**: Fosters a sacred and calming environment.

9. Ginkgo Biloba Tea for Focus

- **Ingredients**: 1 tsp dried ginkgo leaves, 1 cup boiling water.
- **Method**: Steep for 10 minutes, strain, and drink before mindfulness exercises.
- **Benefits**: Improves mental clarity and sharpens focus.

10. Sacred Space with Herbal Sachets

- **Ingredients**: Dried lavender, chamomile, and rosemary, small fabric pouch.
- **Method**: Place herbs in a pouch and keep it near your meditation cushion.
- **Benefits**: Encourages relaxation and grounds your energy.

11. Holy Basil and Ashwagandha Adaptogenic Tea

- **Ingredients**: 1/2 tsp holy basil powder, 1/2 tsp ashwagandha powder, 1 cup hot water.
- **Method**: Mix powders in hot water, stir well, and drink before meditating.
- **Benefits**: Reduces stress and fosters mental stillness.

12. Rose Quartz Meditation Practice

- **Practice**: Hold a rose quartz crystal during meditation, focusing on self-love and compassion.
- **Benefits**: Promotes emotional balance and spiritual connection.

13. Jasmine and Chamomile Pillow for Restful Meditation

- **Ingredients**: Dried jasmine flowers, dried chamomile, small fabric pouch.
- **Method**: Fill the pouch and place it near your meditation space.
- **Benefits**: Enhances tranquility and mental focus.

14. Reishi Mushroom Tea for Grounding

- **Ingredients**: 1 tsp reishi mushroom powder, 1 cup boiling water.
- **Method**: Steep for 15 minutes, strain, and drink before mindfulness practices.
- **Benefits**: Grounds energy and promotes spiritual clarity.

15. Rosemary and Eucalyptus Room Spray

- **Ingredients**: 1/2 cup distilled water, 5 drops rosemary essential oil, 5 drops eucalyptus oil, spray bottle.
- **Method**: Mix and spritz the air around your meditation space.
- **Benefits**: Invigorates the senses and sharpens focus.

16. Candlelight Trataka (Meditative Gazing)

- **Practice**: Light a candle and gaze at the flame for 5–10 minutes, allowing the mind to settle.
- **Benefits**: Enhances focus and calms racing thoughts.

17. Adaptogenic Meditation Tonic

- **Ingredients**: 1 tsp schisandra berry powder, 1 cup warm water.
- **Method**: Mix and sip during meditation preparation.
- **Benefits**: Supports stamina and resilience during prolonged meditative sessions.

18. Sound Healing with Herbal Infusion

- **Practice**: Drink holy basil or chamomile tea while using a Tibetan singing bowl or listening to meditative sounds.
- **Benefits**: Aligns mental and emotional energy for deeper mindfulness.

19. Lemon Balm Tea for Emotional Balance

- **Ingredients**: 1 tsp dried lemon balm, 1 cup boiling water.
- **Method**: Steep for 10 minutes, strain, and drink.
- **Benefits**: Calms emotions and prepares the mind for meditation.

20. Yoga Nidra with Tulsi Tea

- **Ingredients**: 1 tsp dried tulsi leaves, 1 cup boiling water.
- **Method**: Sip the tea and then lie down to practice Yoga Nidra (guided relaxation).

- **Benefits**: Deepens relaxation and spiritual renewal.

21. Herbal Foot Bath for Grounding

- **Ingredients**: 1/4 cup dried rosemary, 1/4 cup dried lavender, warm water.
- **Method**: Add herbs to warm water and soak feet before meditation.
- **Benefits**: Grounds energy and relaxes the body.

22. Peppermint and Rosemary Focus Balm

- **Ingredients**: 2 tbsp coconut oil, 5 drops peppermint oil, 5 drops rosemary oil.
- **Method**: Mix oils and apply to your temples before mindfulness exercises.
- **Benefits**: Clears the mind and enhances focus.

23. Guided Meditation with Frankincense Oil

- **Ingredients**: 5 drops frankincense essential oil, a diffuser.
- **Method**: Diffuse oil during a guided meditation session.
- **Benefits**: Promotes spiritual clarity and deepens meditative states.

24. Lemon and Mint Inhalation for Refreshing Focus

- **Ingredients**: 1 slice fresh lemon, 1 tsp dried mint, bowl of hot water.
- **Method**: Place ingredients in hot water, cover your head with a towel, and inhale deeply for 5 minutes.
- **Benefits**: Clears mental fog and enhances mindfulness.

25. Lavender and Valerian Restorative Tea

- **Ingredients**: 1 tsp dried lavender, 1/2 tsp dried valerian root, 1 cup boiling water.
- **Method**: Steep for 10 minutes, strain, and drink before bedtime meditation.
- **Benefits**: Promotes calmness and prepares the mind for restorative meditation.

1. Daily Herbal Renewal Tea Blend

- **Ingredients**: 1 tsp holy basil, 1 tsp nettle leaves, 1 tsp dried lemon balm, 1 cup boiling water.
- **Method**: Steep all ingredients in boiling water for 10 minutes. Sip in the morning to start the day fresh.
- **Benefits**: Cleanses the body, restores vitality, and supports mental clarity.

2. The 3-Day Cleansing Tonic

- **Ingredients**: 1 tsp grated ginger, 1 tsp fresh lemon juice, 1 tsp raw honey, 1 cup warm water.
- **Method**: Drink this tonic every morning for three days while journaling about what you're letting go of.
- **Benefits**: Clears the digestive system while focusing on emotional and spiritual renewal.

3. Hands-in-Soil Practice

- **Practice**: Spend 10 minutes a week tending to a plant or herb in your garden or a potted plant in your home.
- **Benefits**: Grounds your energy and connects you to the earth's renewing power.

4. Holy Basil and Mint Bath Soak

- **Ingredients**: 1/4 cup dried holy basil, 1/4 cup dried mint, 1/2 cup Epsom salt.
- **Method**: Add ingredients to warm bathwater, soak for 20 minutes, and focus on releasing negativity.
- **Benefits**: Detoxifies the body and calms the mind.

5. Herbal Oil Massage for Cleansing Energy

- **Ingredients**: 1/4 cup sesame oil, 5 drops lavender essential oil, 5 drops rosemary essential oil.
- **Method**: Warm the oil and massage it onto your body before showering. Wash it off with warm water.
- **Benefits**: Releases toxins and stagnant energy stored in the body.

6. Detox Soup for Physical and Emotional Cleansing

- **Ingredients**: 1 cup chopped dandelion greens, 1/2 cup chopped kale, 1 tsp turmeric, vegetable broth.
- **Method**: Simmer all ingredients for 15 minutes. Eat mindfully, focusing on nourishment.
- **Benefits**: Supports the liver and digestive system while symbolizing emotional cleansing.

7. Dandelion Root Tea for Liver Detox

- **Ingredients**: 1 tsp dried dandelion root, 1 cup boiling water.
- **Method**: Simmer the dandelion root for 10 minutes, strain, and drink before bedtime.
- **Benefits**: Supports liver function and gently detoxifies the body.

8. Rosemary and Sage Smoke Cleansing

- **Ingredients**: 1 bundle of dried rosemary and sage.
- **Method**: Light the bundle and allow the smoke to waft through your home or around your body.
- **Benefits**: Clears stagnant energy and renews your environment.

9. Warm Herbal Compress for Emotional Release

- **Ingredients**: 1 tbsp dried chamomile, 1 tbsp dried lavender, 1 bowl of hot water, a soft cloth.
- **Method**: Steep the herbs in hot water, soak the cloth, and place it over your heart or forehead for 10 minutes.
- **Benefits**: Releases emotional tension and promotes relaxation.

10. Cleansing Green Smoothie

- **Ingredients**: 1 cup spinach, 1/2 cucumber, 1/2 apple, 1 tsp spirulina, 1 cup water.
- **Method**: Blend all ingredients until smooth and drink as a mid-morning refreshment.
- **Benefits**: Flushes toxins while restoring vitality.

11. Nettle and Ginger Hair Rinse

- **Ingredients**: 1/2 cup nettle tea, 1 slice fresh ginger.
- **Method**: Brew nettle tea with ginger, let it cool, and use it as a final hair rinse after washing.
- **Benefits**: Cleanses the scalp and refreshes your energy field.

12. Write a Cleansing Intention List

- **Practice**: Write a list of habits, thoughts, or emotions you're ready to release. Keep it as a reminder of your commitment to renewal.
- **Benefits**: Tangibly acknowledges what you're letting go of.

13. Lemon Balm and Mint Morning Infusion

- **Ingredients**: 1 tsp dried lemon balm, 1 tsp dried mint, 1 cup boiling water.
- **Method**: Steep and sip this infusion first thing in the morning.
- **Benefits**: Clears mental fog and refreshes the spirit.

14. Weekly Gratitude Ritual with Lavender Tea

- **Ingredients**: 1 tsp dried lavender, 1 cup boiling water.
- **Method**: Brew tea and sip slowly while writing down one thing you're grateful for each day of the week.
- **Benefits**: Creates a cycle of positivity and emotional cleansing.

15. Mint and Lemon Foot Soak

- **Ingredients**: 1/4 cup Epsom salt, 5 fresh mint leaves, juice of 1/2 lemon.
- **Method**: Add ingredients to warm water and soak your feet for 15 minutes.
- **Benefits**: Releases built-up tension and refreshes your energy.

16. Herbal Detox Stew

- **Ingredients**: 1/2 cup chopped carrots, 1/2 cup chopped celery, 1 tsp dried thyme, 1 tsp turmeric, vegetable broth.
- **Method**: Simmer all ingredients for 20 minutes and eat slowly.
- **Benefits**: Cleanses the body and nourishes the soul.

17. Rosemary Hair Massage Oil

- **Ingredients**: 1/4 cup coconut oil, 5 drops rosemary essential oil.
- **Method**: Warm the oil and massage it into your scalp before washing.
- **Benefits**: Revitalizes the scalp and symbolizes clearing mental clutter.

18. The Daily Reset with Chamomile Tea

- **Ingredients**: 1 tsp dried chamomile, 1 cup boiling water.

- **Method**: Brew and sip slowly in the evening, reflecting on your day and letting go of tension.
- **Benefits**: Calms the mind and closes the day with clarity.

19. Simple Water Offering Ritual

- **Practice**: Pour a small cup of water outdoors while saying, "I return this water with gratitude and release what I no longer need."
- **Benefits**: Symbolizes letting go and spiritual cleansing.

20. Gratitude Stone Practice

- **Ingredients**: A small, smooth stone.
- **Method**: Hold the stone each morning and state one thing you're grateful for before placing it back in its spot.
- **Benefits**: Grounds your day in positivity and mindfulness.

21. Morning Reflection with Peppermint Tea

- **Ingredients**: 1 tsp dried peppermint, 1 cup boiling water.
- **Method**: Brew and drink while reflecting on one positive thought for the day ahead.
- **Benefits**: Encourages mindful focus and freshness.

22. Holy Basil Night Ritual

- **Ingredients**: 1 tsp dried holy basil, 1 cup boiling water.
- **Method**: Brew and sip slowly before bedtime, reflecting on one lesson from the day.
- **Benefits**: Grounds the spirit and prepares you for restful sleep.

23. Cleansing Hair Rinse with Apple Cider Vinegar

- **Ingredients**: 1/4 cup apple cider vinegar, 1 cup water.
- **Method**: Use as a final rinse after washing your hair.
- **Benefits**: Clears buildup and refreshes your energy.

24. Gentle Movement Practice

- **Practice**: Spend 5 minutes each morning stretching or practicing slow movements like tai chi.
- **Benefits**: Encourages energy flow and physical renewal.

25. Mint and Lemon Skin Toner

- **Ingredients**: 1/4 cup mint tea, juice of 1/4 lemon.
- **Method**: Dab onto your skin with a cotton pad after cleansing.
- **Benefits**: Refreshes and cleanses the skin while symbolizing renewal.

Part IV: Beyond the Basics

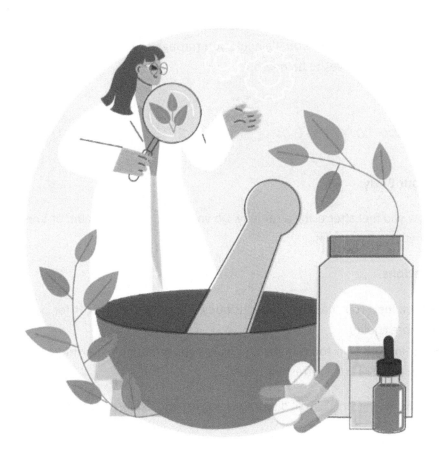

"To go beyond is to dive deeper—not into complexity, but into simplicity understood profoundly."

– Lao Tzu

4.1 Tailoring Remedies to Your Needs

As someone who's spent years blending ancient Ayurvedic wisdom with the realities of modern life, I've learned one thing: healing is personal. No two people are the same. What works for one person might not work as effectively for another. Our bodies are unique, shaped by our experiences, environments, and needs.

In this chapter, we'll explore how to customize remedies, tune into your body's responses, and refine your approach to find what truly works for you. I'll guide you through the art of customizing herbal remedies, because your body's voice deserves to be heard.

1. Listening to Your Body: The First Step in Customization

The Wisdom of Your Body:

Pay attention to how you feel after using a remedy. Do you feel energized, calm, or uneasy? These signals guide you toward better adjustments.

Examples of Variations:

- If a ginger tea feels too "heating" for your body, consider swapping it for peppermint or fennel, which are more cooling.
- If a lavender-infused oil is too calming and makes you lethargic, experiment with adding a drop of rosemary essential oil for a refreshing boost.

Pro Tip: Don't just stop at the first sign of discomfort. Adjust and explore. Herbs are flexible allies.

2. How to Adjust Recipes Based on Preferences and Symptoms

Adjusting Flavor Profiles:

- **For Bitter Tastes**: Add a bit of honey or licorice root to soften the flavor of remedies like dandelion or nettle tea.
- **For Spicy Remedies**: If remedies like turmeric or ginger feel too strong, dilute with more water or pair with soothing herbs like chamomile or mint.

Adjusting Strength and Potency:

- **Start Low and Go Slow**: Begin with smaller doses, especially if you're new to an herb or remedy. Increase gradually as you observe your body's response.

Pro Tip: Think of potency like seasoning in cooking—it's easier to add more than to take it out.

Adjusting for Specific Symptoms:

Example 1: Headaches

- Start with a base of peppermint tea for its cooling properties.
- Add a pinch of dried rosemary if the headache feels tension-based.
- Swap peppermint for ginger if the headache is tied to indigestion.

Example 2: Digestive Issues

- **Base Recipe:** Fennel tea for bloating.
- **Adjustments:** Add chamomile for calming the digestive tract, or ginger for nausea.

"Your remedy should feel like it's speaking directly to your needs. If it feels generic, tweak it. Herbs thrive in dialogue, not monologue."

3. Journaling to Track Your Journey

Keeping a journal is one of the most powerful tools for tailoring remedies to your needs. It allows you to document what works, what doesn't, and how you feel after each remedy.

What to Include in Your Journal:

- **The Remedy**: Write down the recipe you used, including the quantities and preparation method.
- **Your Symptoms**: Note what you were trying to address (e.g., anxiety, headache, indigestion).
- **Your Response**: How did you feel after taking the remedy? Was it effective? Did you notice side effects?
- **Adjustments Made**: If you adjusted the recipe (e.g., reducing ginger or adding peppermint), record those changes.
- **Observations Over Time**: Track patterns over days or weeks to identify long-term effects.

Sample Journal Entry:

- **Date**: March 5, 2024
- **Remedy**: Lemon balm and lavender tea (1 tsp lemon balm, 1/2 tsp lavender, 1 cup boiling water).

- **Symptoms**: Evening stress and racing thoughts.
- **Response**: Felt calmer within 20 minutes but also slightly drowsy.
- **Adjustments**: Next time, reduce lavender to 1/4 tsp to avoid feeling too sleepy.

4. Common Adjustments Based on Sensitivities

For People Sensitive to Strong Tastes:

- Use milder herbs as a base (e.g., chamomile or lemon balm) and gradually add more potent herbs like ginger or turmeric.

For Digestive Sensitivities:

- Reduce "hot" herbs like cayenne or ginger and replace with gentler options like fennel or cardamom.

For Sleep Issues

- Start with calming herbs like chamomile or passionflower. If they're not strong enough, add valerian root or a drop of ashwagandha tincture.

5. The Importance of Patience

The Slow Medicine Philosophy:

Herbal remedies don't work like pharmaceuticals. Their effects are often gentle and cumulative. Be patient with the process and don't be afraid to refine as you go.

My Reflection:

One of my first friend came to me with a deep distrust of natural remedies. She expected immediate results, and when chamomile didn't soothe her stress in one night, she gave up. But when she returned weeks later, I asked her to combine chamomile with holy basil and to journal her experience. A month later, she told me she'd finally found her calm. It wasn't just the remedy—it was the commitment to listening to her body.

6. Creating Your Personalized Remedy Toolbox

Over time, you'll notice certain herbs or combinations work best for you. These become your "go-to" remedies for specific issues.

Example:

- **For Sleep:** Chamomile + lemon balm (with lavender if stress is high).
- **For Digestive Relief:** Fennel + peppermint (ginger for nausea).
- **For Stress Relief:** Holy basil + passionflower (with a pinch of cinnamon for warmth).

Pro Tip: Your toolbox is as unique as your fingerprint. Build it with care, and it will become your lifelong ally.

Herbal healing isn't a rigid science—it's an art, guided by intuition, experience, and self-awareness. By tailoring remedies to your needs and staying curious about how your body responds, you'll develop a deeper relationship with plants and yourself. Trust the process, and let it unfold naturally.

4.2 Foraging for Wild Herbs

Foraging is an ancient practice that connects us deeply with the earth. Gathering wild herbs not only provides fresh, potent ingredients for remedies but also deepens your relationship with nature. However, foraging is more than just picking plants—it's about doing so with respect, knowledge, and a deep sense of responsibility.

Ethical Foraging Practices: What to Pick, What to Leave

The Principles of Ethical Foraging:

- **Take Only What You Need**: Never harvest more than 10% of a plant population in one area. This ensures the plant can regrow and thrive.
- **Know Your Plants**: Positive identification is crucial—many plants have toxic look-alikes. When in doubt, leave it be.
- **Harvest Responsibly**:
  - Leave enough for pollinators and wildlife.
  - Avoid damaging roots or disturbing the surrounding environment.
- **Avoid Polluted Areas**: Do not forage near busy roads, industrial areas, or sprayed fields.
- **Respect Private and Protected Lands**: Always get permission before foraging on private property, and avoid foraging in protected or conservation areas unless allowed.
- **Leave the Area Better Than You Found It**: If possible, clean up trash, or spread seeds to encourage plant regrowth.

What to Leave Behind:

- **Rare or Endangered Plants**: Some herbs, like wild ginseng or certain orchids, are at risk due to overharvesting. Learn to identify and protect them.
- **Plants That Don't Look Healthy**: Avoid plants covered in mold, pests, or showing signs of disease.
- **Seeds and Roots (When Possible)**: Harvest leaves or flowers and leave seeds and roots so the plant can regenerate.

When I started foraging, I was eager to take everything I recognized. My teacher stopped me and said, 'Pick what you'll use today. The rest belongs to the earth.' That simple advice transformed my practice—it's not about abundance, but balance.

Identifying 10 Common Wild Plants (with Photos and Tips)

Here's a list of ten easy-to-identify wild plants that are beginner-friendly, versatile, and often abundant.

1. Dandelion (Taraxacum officinale)

- **Identification**: Bright yellow flowers, jagged tooth-like leaves, milky sap in the stem.
- **Uses**: Leaves for salads or teas, roots for detoxifying tonics.
- **Foraging Tip**: Best harvested in spring or fall when the leaves are tender and roots are full of nutrients.

2. Plantain (Plantago major/lanceolata)

- **Identification**: Broad or lance-shaped leaves with parallel veins, small green flower spikes.
- **Uses**: Leaves for wound poultices or soothing teas.
- **Foraging Tip**: Found in compacted soils like sidewalks, but forage from cleaner areas.

3. Chickweed (Stellaria media)

- **Identification**: Delicate, star-like white flowers; small oval leaves; grows in mats.
- **Uses**: Cooling teas, skin salves, and edible greens for salads.
- **Foraging Tip**: Harvest in spring before it flowers abundantly.

4. Yarrow (Achillea millefolium)

- **Identification**: Fern-like leaves and flat clusters of tiny white flowers.
- **Uses**: Teas for fever, wound powders, or skin tonics.
- **Foraging Tip**: Often found in meadows or sunny patches. Harvest leaves and flowers in early summer.

5. Wild Mint (Mentha spp.)

- **Identification**: Square stems, strong minty smell, small purple or white flowers.
- **Uses**: Teas, digestive tonics, or infused oils.
- **Foraging Tip**: Look near streams or wet areas. Always confirm it's mint by its scent and square stems.

6. Stinging Nettle (Urtica dioica)

- **Identification**: Jagged, serrated leaves with fine stinging hairs, grows in dense clusters.
- **Uses**: Nutrient-rich teas, soups, and hair rinses.
- **Foraging Tip**: Wear gloves to avoid stings. Harvest in early spring before flowering.

7. Elderberry (Sambucus nigra/canadensis)

- **Identification**: Clusters of small, dark purple berries; serrated leaves with opposite branching; white flower clusters in spring.
- **Uses**: Berries for immune-boosting syrups, flowers for teas or skin tonics.
- **Foraging Tip**: Never eat raw berries—always cook them to neutralize toxins.

8. Red Clover (Trifolium pratense)

- **Identification**: Pink-purple round flower heads, trifoliate leaves often marked with a white crescent.
- **Uses**: Teas for hormonal balance or edible flowers in salads.
- **Foraging Tip**: Harvest flowers in full bloom in summer.

9. Burdock (Arctium lappa)

- **Identification**: Large, heart-shaped leaves and spiny burrs; grows up to 6 feet tall.
- **Uses**: Roots for detoxifying teas and soups.
- **Foraging Tip**: Dig roots in late fall or early spring when energy is concentrated in them.

10. Wild Rose (Rosa spp.)

- **Identification**: Thorny stems, fragrant five-petaled pink flowers, and round rose hips in autumn.
- **Uses**: Rose hips for vitamin C-rich teas, petals for infused oils or soothing skin masks.
- **Foraging Tip**: Harvest rose hips after the first frost for maximum potency.

Seasonal Foraging Calendar

Spring (March-May)

- **Best Foraged:** Dandelion leaves, stinging nettle, chickweed, plantain.
- **Why:** Plants are young, tender, and full of nutrients after winter.

Summer (June-August)

- **Best Foraged:** Red clover, yarrow, wild mint, elderflowers.
- **Why**: Flowers and aerial parts are at their peak bloom and potency.

Autumn (September-November)

- **Best Foraged:** Elderberries, burdock roots, rose hips, dandelion roots.
- **Why**: Energy returns to the roots, making them most potent.

Winter (December-February)

- **Best Foraged:** Evergreen needles (pine, spruce), bark (in small amounts, like willow for pain relief).
- **Why**: Limited growth above ground, but trees and conifers provide winter support.

Foraging is an act of gratitude as much as it is a skill. Each time you pick a plant, you're participating in an ancient relationship between humans and nature. Remember to approach the earth as a partner, not a resource. The more you honor what you forage, the more the earth will provide for you in return.

4.3 Preserving Herbal Wisdom

Preserving your creations ensures their potency and allows you to share their benefits with others. Whether you're storing remedies for personal use or crafting heartfelt gifts for loved ones, this chapter will guide you through the essentials of proper preservation and the joy of sharing herbal wisdom.

How to Store Remedies for Long-Term Use

Proper storage ensures the freshness, potency, and safety of your herbal remedies. Here's how to handle different types of preparations:

1. Infusions and Decoctions

Shelf Life: 1–3 days (if refrigerated).

Storage Tips:

- Store in a glass jar with a tight lid in the refrigerator.
- Add a label with the name, ingredients, and date of preparation.
- For longer storage, freeze in ice cube trays and thaw as needed.

Pro Tip: Infusions and decoctions are best made fresh. To avoid waste, prepare small batches—just enough for a day or two.

2. Tinctures

Shelf Life: Up to 5 years (if stored properly).

Storage Tips:

- Keep in amber or dark glass bottles to protect from light.
- Store in a cool, dark place (like a cabinet or pantry).
- Use airtight droppers or lids to prevent evaporation.

Labeling: Include the herb name, extraction medium (e.g., alcohol or glycerin), and date of preparation. Example: "Echinacea Tincture, Vodka Base, May 2024."

3. Powders

Shelf Life: 6–12 months (depending on freshness of the herbs).

Storage Tips:

- Store in airtight glass jars or food-safe tins.
- Use silica gel packets or a small muslin bag of rice to absorb moisture.
- Keep away from heat and sunlight to prevent degradation.

Labeling: Include the name of the herb, preparation date, and suggested use (e.g., "Ashwagandha Powder: Add 1 tsp to warm milk").

4. Salves and Balms

Shelf Life: 6–12 months (depending on the carrier oil and preservatives used).

Storage Tips:

- Use tins or small glass jars with tight lids.
- Store in a cool, dry place (balms may melt in high heat).
- Optional: Add a few drops of vitamin E oil to extend shelf life.

Labeling: Include the intended use, ingredients, and any precautions (e.g., "Calendula Salve: For minor cuts and rashes. Contains beeswax—avoid if allergic.").

5. Dried Herbs

Shelf Life: 1–2 years (depending on how they're stored).

Storage Tips:

- Use glass jars with airtight lids to keep out moisture.
- Store in a dark, cool place to prevent light and heat damage.
- Check periodically for signs of mold or discoloration.

Labeling: Include the herb name, date of drying, and origin (e.g., "Dried Mint: Homegrown, August 2024").

6. Syrups

Shelf Life: 1–2 months (refrigerated).

Storage Tips:

- Use sterilized glass bottles or jars.
- Optional: Add a splash of vodka to the syrup as a natural preservative.

Labeling: Note the herb name, date of preparation, and storage instructions (e.g., "Elderberry Syrup: Refrigerate and use by March 2024.").

Properly Labeling Your Creations for Safety and Convenience

Why Labeling Matters:

- **Safety**: Avoid accidental misuse by clearly identifying contents and any potential allergens.
- **Convenience**: Easily find remedies when you need them.
- **Sharing**: Well-labeled remedies make thoughtful and safe gifts.

What to Include on a Label:

- Name of the remedy (e.g., "Chamomile and Lavender Sleep Tea").
- Ingredients (especially for those with allergies).
- Preparation date and expiration date.
- Instructions for use (e.g., "Steep 1 tsp in hot water for 10 minutes").
- Any precautions or warnings (e.g., "Not recommended during pregnancy").

Creative Labeling Ideas:

- Use kraft paper labels for a rustic look or colorful washi tape for a playful touch.
- Write with waterproof pens to prevent smudging.
- Use small chalkboard tags tied with twine for reusable jars.

Preserving Herbal Wisdom and Passing It On

Preserving your herbal remedies is more than just ensuring their longevity—it's about creating a bridge between the wisdom of nature and your daily life. When you take the time to carefully store and label your creations, you're honoring the care and intention that went into their making. Each jar of tincture, bottle of infused oil, or pouch of dried herbs becomes a tangible expression of your connection with the earth.

But there's another layer to this practice: the joy of sharing. Just as herbs have been passed down through generations—taught from one healer to the next—you, too, carry the responsibility and privilege of being a steward of this knowledge. Whether it's gifting a calming tea blend to a stressed friend, offering an elderberry syrup during cold season, or simply sharing a story about how a remedy worked for you, every act of giving spreads the healing power of nature.

Herbal wisdom thrives when it's shared. When you open your heart and your practice to others, you're not only helping those around you—you're ensuring that this ancient knowledge continues to grow and flourish in our modern world. So as you preserve your remedies, remember this: you're not just keeping them for yourself; you're cultivating a legacy of healing, care, and connection that can ripple outward in ways you might not yet see.

Part V: Resources for the Modern Herbalist

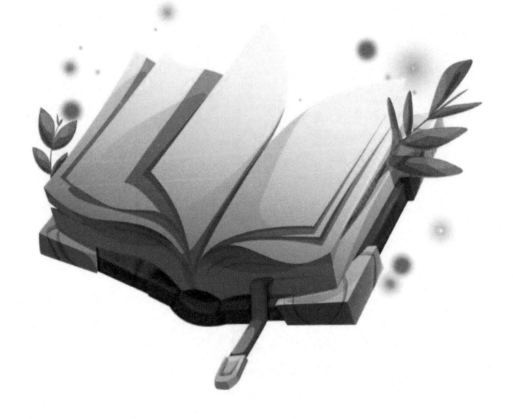

"Herbs have been our allies since the beginning of time. All we need to do is remember."

5.1 Common Herb Profiles: A Quick Reference

Herb	Medicinal Properties	Uses
Chamomile	Calming, anti-inflammatory, digestive aid	Relieves stress, soothes upset stomach, promotes sleep
Peppermint	Antispasmodic, digestive aid, cooling	Eases nausea, relieves headaches, soothes bloating
Ginger	Anti-nausea, anti-inflammatory, warming	Reduces nausea, supports digestion, alleviates joint pain
Holy Basil (Tulsi)	Adaptogenic, calming, immune-boosting	Reduces stress, balances energy, enhances immunity
Lavender	Relaxing, antiseptic, anti-inflammatory	Calms anxiety, soothes headaches, promotes restful sleep
Dandelion	Detoxifying, diuretic, liver-supportive	Cleanses the liver, aids digestion, reduces water retention
Nettle	Mineral-rich, anti-inflammatory, detoxifying	Supports energy, reduces allergies, strengthens hair and nails
Elderberry	Antiviral, immune-boosting, antioxidant	Fights colds and flu, boosts immunity, protects cells
Yarrow	Astringent, anti-inflammatory, fever-reducing	Stops minor bleeding, reduces fevers, soothes rashes
Calendula	Wound-healing, anti-inflammatory, antimicrobial	Heals cuts, soothes skin irritation, supports digestion
Fennel	Digestive aid, carminative, anti-spasmodic	Relieves bloating, aids digestion, soothes cramps
Lemon Balm	Calming, antiviral, digestive aid	Reduces anxiety, supports sleep, soothes cold sores
Rosemary	Stimulating, antioxidant, anti-inflammatory	Enhances memory, improves circulation, reduces joint pain
Thyme	Antimicrobial, expectorant, antioxidant	Relieves coughs, fights infections, supports digestion
Sage	Antimicrobial, memory-enhancing, astringent	Soothes sore throats, improves focus, balances hormones
Echinacea	Immune-boosting, antimicrobial, anti-inflammatory	Prevents colds, fights infections, reduces inflammation
Red Clover	Hormone-balancing, detoxifying, anti-inflammatory	Eases menopausal symptoms, supports detoxification
Ashwagandha	Adaptogenic, calming, stress-reducing	Reduces anxiety, balances energy, supports adrenal health
Turmeric	Anti-inflammatory, antioxidant, pain-relieving	Reduces joint pain, supports digestion, boosts skin health
Plantain	Wound-healing, anti-inflammatory, soothing	Treats minor cuts, soothes skin rashes, calms bites and stings

5.2 Herbal Energetics Chart

Energetic Quality	Description	Examples of Herbs
Warming	Stimulates circulation, boosts metabolism, dispels cold sensations; ideal for cold or stagnant conditions.	Ginger, Cinnamon, Black Pepper, Garlic, Cayenne, Clove
Cooling	Soothes inflammation, calms heat or irritation; ideal for hot, feverish, or overactive conditions.	Peppermint, Chamomile, Lemon Balm, Dandelion, Aloe Vera
Drying	Reduces excess moisture or mucus; ideal for damp conditions like colds with congestion.	Sage, Thyme, Yarrow, Horsetail, Nettle
Moistening	Replenishes dryness, soothes tissues, hydrates; ideal for dry skin, throat, or digestion.	Marshmallow Root, Licorice, Slippery Elm, Oatstraw

How to Use This Chart:

1. **Identify the Energetic Imbalance**: For example, if you're experiencing a cold and sluggish digestion, choose warming herbs. If your throat feels dry and scratchy, opt for moistening herbs.
2. **Customize Remedies**: Blend herbs with complementary energetics (e.g., warming ginger with cooling lemon balm for balanced relief).
3. **Adjust Over Time**: As conditions shift, adapt your choice of herbs to suit evolving needs.

5.3 Herbal Log: A sample template for tracking herbal remedies, symptoms, and results

Keeping track of your herbal remedies is key to understanding what works best for your body. The **Herbal Log** helps you document the remedies you try, the symptoms you address, and the results you experience over time.

By tracking your journey, you'll gain valuable insights into your unique needs, allowing you to refine dosages, experiment with combinations, and recognize patterns that support your health. This simple yet powerful tool transforms your herbal practice into a personalized roadmap for wellness.

Date	Remedy Used	Dosage/Method	Purpose/Sympt om	Immediate Effects	Long-Term Results	Notes/Adjustme nts
MM/DD/YYYY	Exampler Chamomile Tea	1 tsp dried chamomile steeped in 1 cup hot water, 2x daily	Stress and difficulty sleeping	Felt calm within 20 minutes	Improved sleep quality over a week	Reduce to 1x daily for less drowsiness

Date	Remedy Used	Dosage/Method	Purpose/Sympt om	Immediate Effects	Long-Term Results	Notes/Adjustme nts

Before We Part

As we close the final pages of this book, I want to extend my deepest gratitude to you for joining me on this journey into the world of forgotten home apothecary. This has been more than a writing project for me—it has been a labor of love, a blending of research, personal exploration, and an unshakable belief in the healing power of nature.

Every remedy, every insight, and every piece of wisdom shared here was carefully compiled with the hope that it will inspire you, empower you, and help you take your first or next steps into herbal healing. It is my wish that these pages not only guide you in crafting remedies but also rekindle a connection to the earth and its boundless gifts.

Herbalism is a path of discovery. As you try these remedies, tailor them to your needs, and pass them on to others, I hope you'll find as much joy and fulfillment as I have in creating and sharing this book with you.

Before we part ways, I'd love to hear about your experiences with this book. Did it help you? Inspire you? Offer something new? Your honest reviews mean the world to me—they not only help me grow as an author but also allow this knowledge to reach and benefit others like you.

And finally, remember to have fun! Let the process of healing and learning be as light and natural as the remedies themselves. Every sip of tea, every jar of salve, and every tincture you create is a step toward a deeper connection with yourself and the world around you.

With all my gratitude and encouragement,

Rohit 😊

Amazon Review Link

Glossary

A. Types of Herbal Preparations

- **Decoction**: A method of extracting active ingredients from tough plant materials like roots, bark, and seeds by boiling them in water for an extended period.
- **Infusion**: A water-based preparation where delicate plant parts, such as leaves or flowers, are steeped in hot water (like tea).
- **Tincture**: A concentrated herbal extract made by soaking herbs in alcohol or glycerin to extract and preserve their active compounds.
- **Syrup**: A sweetened herbal preparation made by combining a decoction or infusion with honey or sugar, often used for colds and sore throats.
- **Salve**: A semi-solid preparation made by mixing herbal oils with beeswax, used externally for skin conditions or pain relief.
- **Poultice**: A paste made from mashed herbs or powders applied directly to the skin for healing wounds, inflammation, or infections.
- **Compress**: A cloth soaked in an herbal infusion or decoction, applied to the skin to soothe inflammation or reduce swelling.
- **Oxymel**: A blend of vinegar, honey, and herbs, often used for respiratory health and as a digestive tonic.
- **Capsules**: Dried, powdered herbs encapsulated in pill form for easy ingestion.
- **Liniment**: An alcohol- or oil-based preparation applied to the skin for muscle aches or pain relief.

B. Common Herbal Actions

- **Adaptogen**: Herbs that help the body adapt to stress and maintain balance, such as ashwagandha or holy basil.
- **Anti-inflammatory**: Herbs that reduce inflammation, such as turmeric or ginger.
- **Antimicrobial**: Herbs that fight bacteria, viruses, or fungi, such as thyme or garlic.
- **Astringent**: Herbs that tighten and tone tissues, often used for wounds or oily skin, such as yarrow or witch hazel.
- **Carminative**: Herbs that soothe the digestive system and reduce gas or bloating, such as fennel or peppermint.
- **Demulcent**: Herbs that soothe and coat irritated tissues, often used for sore throats, such as slippery elm or marshmallow root.

- **Diuretic**: Herbs that increase urine production to help the body eliminate excess fluids, such as dandelion or parsley.
- **Expectorant**: Herbs that loosen mucus and support its expulsion from the respiratory system, such as mullein or licorice root.
- **Nervine**: Herbs that calm the nervous system and support emotional well-being, such as chamomile or lemon balm.

C. Herbal Properties by Energetics

- **Warming Herbs**: Stimulate circulation and boost energy, such as cinnamon or cayenne.
- **Cooling Herbs**: Soothe heat and inflammation, such as peppermint or aloe vera.
- **Drying Herbs**: Reduce excess moisture or mucus, such as sage or horsetail.
- **Moistening Herbs**: Hydrate and soothe dry tissues, such as marshmallow root or licorice.

D. Basic Herbal Tools and Techniques

- **Mortar and Pestle**: A traditional tool used to grind or crush herbs into powders or pastes.
- **Double Boiler**: A tool for gently heating oils and herbs without direct heat, often used for making salves.
- **Amber Glass Bottles**: Used to store tinctures and oils, protecting them from light degradation.
- **Muslin Bag**: A reusable cloth bag used to strain herbal preparations like infusions or decoctions.
- **Infuser**: A device for steeping herbs in water, commonly used for tea preparation.

E. Key Herbal Ingredients and Terms

- **Carrier Oil**: A base oil (such as olive, coconut, or almond oil) used to dilute essential oils or infuse herbs for salves and massage oils.
- **Essential Oil**: Highly concentrated plant extracts used for aromatherapy, requiring dilution before skin application.
- **Beeswax**: A natural wax used to thicken herbal salves or balms.
- **Herbal Vinegar**: A preparation made by infusing vinegar with herbs, often used for digestion or hair rinses.
- **Raw Honey**: Unprocessed honey with natural enzymes, often used in syrups and for wound healing.

F. Herbal Safety and Use

- **Contraindications**: Situations where an herb should not be used, such as during pregnancy or with specific medications.
- **Patch Test**: A method for testing potential skin reactions by applying a small amount of a remedy to a patch of skin.
- **Dosage**: The recommended quantity of an herb or remedy to be used safely and effectively.

G. Seasonal and Foraging Terms

- **Seasonal Foraging**: Harvesting herbs at their peak season for maximum potency (e.g., spring for tender greens like nettle).
- **Wildcrafting**: The practice of harvesting herbs from their natural habitat, done ethically and sustainably.
- **Endangered Plants**: Herbs that are at risk of overharvesting and should be avoided or grown sustainably, such as wild ginseng.

H. Spiritual and Energetic Practices

- **Grounding**: A practice of connecting with the earth to balance energy, often paired with herbal teas like dandelion or nettle.
- **Ritual Use of Herbs**: Incorporating herbs like sage or frankincense into spiritual practices for cleansing or meditation.
- **Affirmation Rituals**: Using herbs like holy basil or lavender alongside affirmations to support emotional healing.

Notes

Notes

Made in the USA
Las Vegas, NV
08 December 2024

13592862R00131